When Your Doctor Says

Heart Disease

D1534673

When Your Doctor Says

Heart Disease

A Guide to Regaining Control
over Your Health and Well-Being

Edited by David A. Cooke, MD, FACP

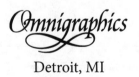

Detroit, MI

Bibliographic Note

This book contains original material as well as material excerpted, adapted, and reprinted from other sources. Complete citations are given at the end of each chapter.

David A. Cooke, MD, FACP, *Editor*
Daniel Hayes, MD, *Contributing Editor*

Wordwright, LLC, *Managing Editor*
Lisa Bakewell, Sandra J. Judd, Zachary Klimecki,
Laura Larsen, Amy Sutton, *Assistant Editors*
WordCo Indexing Services, Inc., *Indexer*
WhimsyInk, *Design and Prepress*
Front cover image © iStockphoto.com/Nigel Silcock
Background illustration © iStockphoto.com/Ali Mazraie Shadi

Omnigraphics
Matthew P. Barbour, Senior Vice President
Kevin M. Hayes, Operations Manager
Peter E. Ruffner, Publisher

Copyright © 2010 Omnigraphics, Inc. All rights reserved.
ISBN 978-0-7808-1168-3

Library of Congress Cataloging-in-Publication Data

When your doctor says heart disease : a guide to regaining control over your health and well-being / edited by David A. Cooke.
  p. cm. -- (When your doctor says)
  Includes bibliographical references and index.
  ISBN 978-0-7808-1168-3 (pbk. : alk. paper) 1. Heart--Diseases--Popular works. 2. Heart--Diseases--Treatment--Popular works. 3. Heart--Diseases--Prevention--Popular works. I. Cooke, David A.
  RC672.W44 2010
  616.1'2075--dc22

                                                          2010033666

Printed in the United States

Contents

Part Three:
Moving Forward

Introduction

The importance of the heart was known in ancient times even though its function was poorly understood. For thousands of years, people believed it to be the seat of thought and the human soul. Our language reflects this with common phrases like "speaking from the heart" and learning things "by heart." Today, its role in the body is far better understood, but even so, most people know little about their heart until a problem develops.

Heart disease is one of the most common serious medical problems in the United States, and it is the leading cause of death. More than 26 million Americans suffer from heart disease. Every year, more than 600,000 people have a first heart attack, and more than 630,000 die from some form of heart disease. Although traditionally considered a male disease, the breadth of heart disease's impact on women is increasingly being recognized.

As a general internal medicine specialist, I spend considerable time working with people with heart disease. Coronary artery disease, heart failure, and heart valve problems are issues I encounter on a daily basis. Having worked with so many people with heart disease, I have seen again and again their desire and need to better understand their medical problems. If you are like them, this book will give you that opportunity.

When Your Doctor Says Heart Disease is intended to help you be an informed patient. It explains the core concepts behind the different forms of heart disease and the terms you may hear during your visits with your doctor. This book also provides details about the treatments for heart disease, and it explains the rationale behind them. There is an extensive discussion about the measures you can take to improve your chances of a good outcome. Finally, there are guides to resources for further education or assistance in treating your disease.

This book is a resource that can reinforce your caregiver's teaching or help answer many of the questions you didn't think to ask at your last doctor's appointment. It is increasingly clear that how your disease is treated determines your life expectancy. Knowing the personal steps you can take will empower you to take control of your disease.

When Your Doctor Says

When Your Doctor Says Heart Disease is part of a series titled *When Your Doctor Says*. The individual books in this series draw on a number of resources, offering you an entire library of accurate and up-to-date information about various medical conditions and their management. The series includes material written by fellow health care professionals and myself as well as information excerpted, adapted, updated, revised, and reprinted from a variety of other organizations, such as various agencies under the National Institutes of Health (NIH), the Centers for Disease Control and Prevention (CDC), and the U. S. Food and Drug Administration (FDA)—sources that are reliable and authoritative but not always efficient at getting information into the hands of the people who need it most.

Omnigraphics, the publisher of the *When Your Doctor Says* books, has a long history of providing health information to consumers. Since 1989, they have published more than 200 volumes in their highly acclaimed *Health Reference Series*, a series of books designed primarily for libraries and library patrons. It has been my pleasure to work with the *Health Reference Series* editors by serving as medical advisor to that project, and I am delighted to have the opportunity to work with them on this endeavor as well.

The books in the *When Your Doctor Says* series expand on the *Health Reference Series* tradition with a special focus on the needs of individual readers. Instead of merely consulting specific sections of a reference book during the confines of a library visit, people can take home and read each *When Your Doctor Says* title at their leisure from cover to cover and refer back to it as often as necessary. The editorial processes that have been developed and that have served for more than 20 years as a trusted means of assembling reliable information form the foundation upon which this series is built. Experienced editors have worked with me to identify, cull, and organize material from a variety of trusted sources. Where it was necessary to fill gaps or provide updated information, I or other qualified individuals and colleagues have written new material. The end result is the book you have in your hands now—a complete and fully indexed resource for people who have been diagnosed with a specific medical condition or who are concerned about a diagnosis in a loved one.

This book, however, is not intended to serve as a tool for diagnosing illness, prescribing treatments, or as a substitute for the physician/patient relationship. All people concerned about medical symptoms or the possibility of disease are encouraged to seek professional care from an appropriate health care provider.

About the Parts of This Book

To ensure easy access to all the information in this book, it is arranged in parts. Each part addresses issues within a specific topical area.

Part One includes information about how the normal heart functions. It also discusses what can go wrong and the many different kinds of heart disease. If you have been recently diagnosed with a heart problem, starting with this part may be the quickest way to find answers to your most pressing questions about your diagnosis.

Part Two explains many of the tests, procedures, and treatments your doctor may order. There has been rapid growth in the number of available cardiac tests and procedures in recent years, and this section will help you understand their uses and limitations. Drug therapy for heart disease has also evolved considerably, and this part discusses the various medications used in treating heart disease. This part will be helpful for new and long-standing patients alike.

Part Three includes actions you can take to help treat your heart disease and improve your heart health. If you're seeking assistance in understanding your care routines, building motivation for continuing your recovery, or preventing or managing complications, the information in this part will help you understand what is required.

Part Four discusses recent heart disease research and how new findings may impact the future for people with heart problems. This part concludes with chapters containing resources for additional help and information.

My Goals for You

I firmly believe educated patients are the best kind of patients. I think this book will teach you what you need to know about your disease and open you to new ideas about how to take the best possible care of yourself. I hope this will help you prepare questions for your doctor and get the most out of your medical visits.

Part One

Understanding Your Diagnosis

The heart is vital to life. Its pumping action circulates blood to carry oxygen and nutrients to all your body's organs and tissues. When things go awry, serious problems result. If you just learned you have a heart problem, you probably have a lot of questions about what caused it and what your diagnosis means. The chapters in this part offer answers.

To begin, we'll look at how the heart and circulatory system work. The first chapter explains heart anatomy, the blood vessels that make up your circulatory system, and the cardiac conduction system—the electrical system that tells your heart when to pump.

The remaining chapters in this part explain some of the most common types of heart disease:

Ischemic heart disease occurs when the blood vessels to the heart are partially or completely blocked. When they are completely blocked, oxygen-rich blood does not reach parts of the heart, and heart muscle dies. This is a heart attack.

Heart failure is a common, but very different, condition. In heart failure, the heart's pumping action does not stop, but it is insufficient to meet the body's needs.

Another problem is related to the rhythm or rate of the heartbeat. If the heart beats too fast, too slow, or irregularly, it is called an arrhythmia. Some arrhythmias don't typically lead to other problems, but other types of arrhythmias can be serious—even life threatening—when they result in insufficient blood flow to the heart, brain, and other organs.

Heart murmurs refer to unusual sounds heard during a heartbeat. Murmurs aren't a disease; they are a symptom of an underlying anomaly in the heart's structure. Many are harmless, but some indicate serious defects in the heart's walls, chambers, or valves. These problems may be congenital (present from birth) or due to damage occurring later in life.

The heart can also be damaged by infections and inflammation. When the endocardium, the inner lining of the heart's chambers and valves, becomes infected, the condition is called infective endocarditis (IE). Inflammation of the pericardium, the membranous sac around the heart, is called pericarditis.

Finally, the heart can be damaged by aortic aneurysms. The aorta is the main artery that carries oxygen-rich blood from the heart to the rest of the body. An aneurysm is a bulge resulting from a weakness in the arterial wall. This can lead to structural changes in the heart, and if the aneurysm breaks open, it can cause life-threatening internal bleeding.

Chapter 1

How the Heart and Circulatory System Work

Your heart is a muscular organ that acts like a pump to continuously send blood throughout your body.

Your heart is at the center of your circulatory system. This system consists of a network of blood vessels, such as arteries, veins, and capillaries. These blood vessels carry blood to and from all areas of your body.

An electrical system regulates your heart and uses electrical signals to contract the heart's walls. When the walls contract, blood is pumped into your circulatory system. A system of inlet and outlet valves in your heart chambers works to ensure blood flows in the right direction.

Your heart is vital to your health and nearly everything that goes on in your body. Without the heart's pumping action, blood can't circulate within your body.

Your blood carries the oxygen and nutrients your organs need to work normally. Blood also carries carbon dioxide, a waste product, to your lungs to be passed out of your body and into the air.

A healthy heart supplies the areas of your body with the right amount of blood at the rate needed to work normally. If disease or injury weakens your heart, your body's organs won't receive enough blood to function normally.

Location and Size

Your heart is located under your rib cage in the center of your chest between your right and left lungs. Its muscular walls beat, or contract, pumping blood continuously to all parts of your body.

The size of your heart can vary depending on your age, size, and the condition of your heart. A normal, healthy, adult heart is generally the size of an average clenched adult fist. Some diseases of the heart can cause it to become larger.

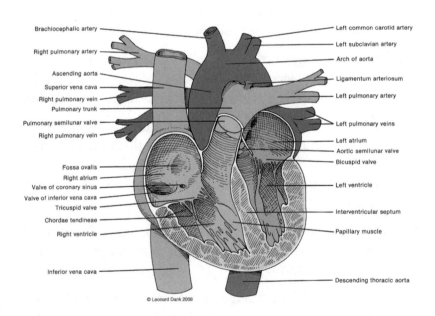

Figure 1.1. Your heart: A cross section.

The Exterior of the Heart

The heart has four chambers: the right and left atria and the right and left ventricles.

Some of the main blood vessels—arteries and veins—that make up your blood circulatory system are directly connected to your heart.

The ventricle on the right side of your heart pumps blood from your heart to your lungs. When you breathe air in, oxygen passes from your lungs through your blood vessels and into your blood. Carbon dioxide, a waste product, is passed from your blood to your lungs through blood vessels and is removed from your body when you breathe out.

The left atrium receives oxygen-rich blood from your lungs. The pumping action of your left ventricle sends this oxygen-rich blood through the aorta (a main artery) to the rest of your body.

The Right Side of Your Heart

The superior and inferior vena cavae are the largest veins in your body.

After your body's organs and tissues have used the oxygen in your blood, the vena cavae carry the oxygen-poor blood back to the right atrium of your heart.

The superior vena cava carries oxygen-poor blood from the upper parts of your body, including your head, chest, arms, and neck. The inferior vena cava carries oxygen-poor blood from the lower parts of your body.

The oxygen-poor blood from the vena cavae flows into your heart's right atrium and then on to the right ventricle. From the right ventricle, the blood is pumped through the pulmonary arteries to your lungs. There, through many small, thin blood vessels called capillaries, the blood picks up more oxygen.

The oxygen-rich blood passes from your lungs back to your heart through the pulmonary veins.

The Left Side of Your Heart

Oxygen-rich blood from your lungs passes through the pulmonary veins. It enters the left atrium and is pumped into the left ventricle. From the left ventricle, the oxygen-rich blood is pumped to the rest of your body through the aorta.

Like all your organs, your heart needs blood rich with oxygen. This oxygen is supplied through the coronary arteries as blood is pumped out of your heart's left ventricle.

Your coronary arteries are located on your heart's surface at the beginning of the aorta. Your coronary arteries carry oxygen-rich blood to all parts of your heart.

The Interior of the Heart

The Septum

The right and left sides of your heart are divided by an internal wall of tissue called the septum. The area of the septum that divides the atria (the two upper chambers of your heart) is called the atrial or interatrial septum.

The area of the septum that divides the ventricles (the two lower chambers of your heart) is called the ventricular or interventricular septum.

Heart Chambers

The heart is divided into four chambers. The two upper chambers of your heart are called atria. The atria receive and collect blood.

The two lower chambers of your heart are called ventricles. The ventricles pump blood out of your heart into your circulatory system to other parts of your body.

Heart Valves

Your heart has four valves. The valves include the aortic valve, the tricuspid valve, the pulmonary valve, and the mitral valve.

Heart Contraction and Blood Flow

Blood Flow

Blood enters the right atrium of your heart from the superior and inferior vena cavae.

From the right atrium, blood is pumped into the right ventricle. From the right ventricle, blood is pumped to your lungs through the pulmonary arteries.

Oxygen-rich blood comes in from your lungs through the pulmonary veins into your heart's left atrium. From the left atrium, the blood is pumped into the left ventricle. The left ventricle pumps the blood to the rest of your body through the aorta.

For the heart to work properly, your blood must flow in only one direction. Your heart's valves make this possible. Both of your heart's ventricles have an in (inlet) valve from the atria and an out (outlet) valve leading to your arteries.

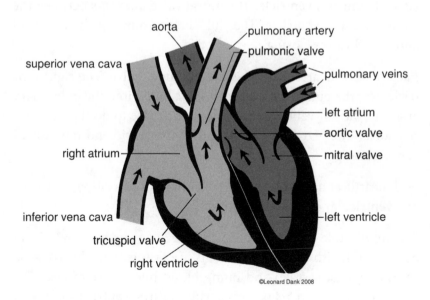

©Leonard Dank 2008

Figure 1.2. Blood flow through the heart.

Healthy valves open and close in very exact coordination with the pumping action of your heart's atria and ventricles. Each valve has a set of flaps—called leaflets or cusps—that seal or open the valves. This allows pumped blood to pass through the chambers and into your arteries without backing up or flowing backward.

Heartbeat

Almost everyone has heard the real or recorded sound of a heartbeat. When your heart beats, it makes a "lub-DUB" sound. Between the time you hear "lub" and "DUB," blood is pumped through your heart and circulatory system.

A heartbeat may seem like a simple, repeated event, but it's a complex series of very precise and coordinated events that take place inside and around your heart.

Each side of your heart uses an inlet valve to move blood between the atrium and ventricle. The tricuspid valve does this between the right atrium and ventricle. The mitral valve does this between the left atrium and ventricle. The "lub" is the sound of the tricuspid and mitral valves closing.

Each of your heart's ventricles has an outlet valve. The right ventricle uses the pulmonary valve to move blood into the pulmonary arteries. The left ventricle uses the aortic valve to do the same for the aorta. The "DUB" is the sound of the aortic and pulmonary valves closing.

Each heartbeat has two basic parts: diastole, or relaxation, and atrial and ventricular systole, or contraction.

During diastole, the atria and ventricles of your heart relax and begin to fill with blood. At the end of diastole, your heart's atria contract (atrial systole) and pump blood into the ventricles. The atria then begin to relax. Next, your heart's ventricles contract (ventricular systole) and pump blood out of your heart.

Pumping Action

Your heart uses its four valves to ensure your blood flows only in one direction. Healthy valves open and close in coordination with the pumping action of your heart's atria and ventricles.

Each valve has a set of flaps called leaflets or cusps. These seal or open the valves, allowing pumped blood to pass through the chambers and into your blood vessels without backing up or flowing backward.

Oxygen-poor blood from the vena cavae fills your heart's right atrium. The atrium contracts (atrial systole). The tricuspid valve located between the right atrium and ventricle opens for a short time and then shuts. This allows blood to enter into the right ventricle without flowing back into the right atrium.

When your heart's right ventricle fills with blood, it contracts (ventricular systole). The pulmonary valve located between your right ventricle and pulmonary artery opens and closes quickly.

This allows blood to enter into your pulmonary arteries without flowing back into the right ventricle. This is important because the right ventricle begins to refill with more blood through the tricuspid valve. Blood travels through the pulmonary arteries to your lungs to pick up oxygen.

Oxygen-rich blood returns from your lungs to your heart's left atrium through the pulmonary veins. As your heart's left atrium fills with blood, it contracts. This event also is called atrial systole.

The mitral valve located between the left atrium and left ventricle opens and closes quickly. This allows blood to pass from the left atrium into the left ventricle without flowing backward.

As the left ventricle fills with blood, it contracts. This event also is called ventricular systole. The aortic valve located between the left ventricle and aorta opens and closes quickly. This allows blood to flow into the aorta. The aorta is the main artery that carries blood from your heart to the rest of your body.

The aortic valve closes quickly to prevent blood from flowing back into the left ventricle, which is already filling up with new blood.

Taking Your Pulse

When your heart pumps blood through your arteries, it creates a pulse that you can feel on the arteries close to the skin's surface. For example, you can feel your pulse on the artery on the underside of your wrist, below your thumb.

You can count how many times your heart beats by taking your pulse. You will need a watch with a second hand.

To find your pulse, gently place your index and middle fingers on the artery located on the inner wrist of either arm, below your thumb. You should feel a pulsing, or tapping, against your fingers.

Watch the second hand and count the number of pulses you feel in 30 seconds. Double that number to find your heart rate, or pulse, for one minute.

The usual resting pulse for an adult is 60 to 100 beats per minute. To find your resting pulse, count your pulse after you have been sitting or resting quietly for at least 10 minutes.

Circulation and Blood Vessels

Your heart and blood vessels make up your overall blood circulatory system. Your blood circulatory system is made up of four subsystems.

Arterial Circulation

Arterial circulation is the part of your overall blood circulatory system that involves arteries, like the aorta and pulmonary arteries.

Arteries are blood vessels that carry blood away from your heart. Healthy arteries are strong and elastic. They become narrow between beats of the heart, and they help keep your blood pressure consistent. This helps blood circulate efficiently through your body.

Arteries branch into smaller blood vessels called arterioles. Arteries and arterioles have strong, flexible walls that allow them to adjust the amount and rate of blood flowing to various parts of your body.

Venous Circulation

Venous circulation is the part of your overall blood circulatory system that involves veins, like the vena cavae and pulmonary veins. Veins are blood vessels that carry blood to your heart.

Veins have thinner walls than arteries. Veins can widen as the amount of blood passing through them increases.

Capillary Circulation

Capillary circulation is the part of your overall blood circulatory system where oxygen, nutrients, and waste pass between your blood and parts of your body.

Capillaries connect the arterial and venous circulatory subsystems. Capillaries are very small blood vessels.

The importance of capillaries lies in their very thin walls. Unlike arteries and veins, capillary walls are thin enough that oxygen and nutrients in your blood can pass through the walls to the parts of your body that need them to work normally.

Capillaries' thin walls also allow waste products like carbon dioxide to pass from your body's organs and tissues into the blood, where it's taken away to your lungs.

Pulmonary Circulation

Pulmonary circulation is the movement of blood from the heart to the lungs and back to the heart again. Pulmonary circulation includes both arterial and venous circulation.

Blood without oxygen is pumped to the lungs from the heart (arterial circulation). Oxygen-rich blood moves from the lungs to the heart through the pulmonary veins (venous circulation).

Pulmonary circulation also includes capillary circulation. Oxygen you breathe in from the air passes through your lungs into your blood through the many capillaries in your lungs. Oxygen-rich blood moves through your pulmonary veins to the left side of your heart and out of the aorta to the rest of your body.

Capillaries in the lungs also remove carbon dioxide from your blood so your lungs can breathe the carbon dioxide out into the air.

Your Heart's Electrical System

Your heart's electrical system controls all the events that occur when your heart pumps blood. The electrical system also is called the cardiac conduction system. If you've ever seen an EKG (electrocardiogram) heart test, you've seen a graphical picture of the heart's electrical activity.

Your heart's electrical system is made up of three main parts:

- The sinoatrial (SA) node, located in the right atrium of your heart

- The atrioventricular (AV) node, located on the interatrial septum close to the tricuspid valve

- The His-Purkinje system, located along the walls of your heart's ventricles

A heartbeat is a complex series of events that take place in your heart. Each beat of your heart is set in motion by an electrical signal from within your heart muscle. In a normal, healthy heart, each beat begins with a signal from the SA node. This is why the SA node is sometimes called your heart's natural pacemaker. Your pulse, or heart rate, is the number of signals the SA node produces per minute.

The signal is generated as the two vena cavae fill your heart's right atrium with blood from other parts of your body. The signal spreads across the cells of your heart's right and left atria. This signal causes the atria to contract, which pushes blood through the open valves from the atria into both ventricles.

The signal arrives at the AV node near the ventricles. It slows for an instant to allow your heart's right and left ventricles to fill with blood. The signal is released and moves along a pathway called the bundle of His, which is located in the walls of your heart's ventricles.

From the bundle of His, the signal fibers divide into left and right bundle branches through the Purkinje fibers, which connect directly to the cells in the walls of your heart's left and right ventricles.

The signal spreads across the cells of your ventricle walls, and both ventricles contract. However, this doesn't happen at exactly the same moment.

The left ventricle contracts an instant before the right ventricle. This pushes blood through the pulmonary valve (for the right ventricle) to your lungs and through the aortic valve (for the left ventricle) to the rest of your body.

As the signal passes, the walls of the ventricles relax and await the next signal.

This process continues over and over as the atria refill with blood and other electrical signals come from the SA node.

Heart Disease

Your heart is made up of many parts working together to pump blood. In a healthy heart, all the parts work well so your heart pumps blood normally. As a result, the parts of your body that depend on the heart to deliver blood also stay healthy.

Heart disease can disrupt a heart's normal electrical system and pumping functions. Diseases and conditions of the heart's muscle make it hard for your heart to pump blood normally.

Damaged or diseased blood vessels make the heart work harder than normal. Problems with the heart's electrical system, called arrhythmias, can make it hard for the heart to pump blood efficiently.

Every year, many men and women in the United States receive a diagnosis of heart disease. Here are some facts about the prevalence and consequences of heart disease in the United States:

- In 2006, 631,636 people died of heart disease. Heart disease caused 26% of deaths—more than one in every four—in the United States.

- Coronary heart disease is the most common type of heart disease. In 2005, 445,687 people died from coronary heart disease.

- Every year, about 785,000 Americans have a first heart attack. Another 470,000 who have already had one or more heart attacks have another attack.

- In 2010, heart disease will cost the United States $316.4 billion. This total includes the cost of health care services, medications, and lost productivity.

Men and Heart Disease

Heart disease is the leading cause of death for men in the United States:

- In 2006, 315,706 men died from heart disease.

- Heart disease killed 26% of men who died in 2006—more than one in every four.

- Heart disease is the leading cause of death for men of most racial/ethnic groups in the United States, including

African Americans, American Indians or Alaska Natives, Hispanics, and whites. For Asian American men, heart disease is second only to cancer.

- In 2006, about 9.4% of white men, 7.8% of black men, and 5.3% of Mexican American men were living with coronary heart disease.

- Half of the men who die suddenly of coronary heart disease have no previous symptoms. Even if you have no symptoms, you may still be at risk for heart disease.

- Between 70% and 89% of sudden cardiac events occur in men.

Women and Heart Disease

Heart disease is also the leading cause of death for women in the United States:

- In 2006, 315,930 women died from heart disease.

- Heart disease killed 26% of women who died in 2006—more than one in every four.

- Although heart disease is sometimes thought of as a man's disease, around the same number of women and men die each year of heart disease in the United States. Unfortunately, 36% of women did not perceive themselves to be at risk for heart disease in a 2005 survey.

- Heart disease is the leading cause of death for women of most racial/ethnic groups in the United States, including African Americans, American Indians or Alaska Natives, Hispanics, and whites. For Asian American women, heart disease is second only to cancer.

- In 2006, about 6.9% of white women, 8.8% of black women, and 6.6% of Mexican American women were living with coronary heart disease.

- Almost two-thirds of women who die suddenly of coronary heart disease have no previous symptoms. Even if you have no symptoms, you may still be at risk for heart disease.

Reviewed for currency and excerpted from "How the Heart Works," National Heart, Lung, and Blood Institute (NHLBI, www.nhlbi.nih.gov), July 2009. Supplemental statistical information is excerpted from "Heart Disease Facts," January 25, 2010, "Men and Heart Disease Fact Sheet," January 27, 2010, and "Women and Heart Disease Fact Sheet," January 27, 2010, all three produced by the Centers for Disease Control and Prevention (CDC, www.cdc.gov).

Chapter 2

Ischemic Heart Disease and Heart Attack

When your coronary arteries are narrowed or blocked due to heart disease, oxygen-rich blood can't reach your heart muscle, which can cause angina or a heart attack.

Angina is chest pain or discomfort that occurs when not enough oxygen-rich blood flows to an area of your heart muscle. A heart attack occurs when blood flow to an area of your heart muscle is completely blocked. This prevents oxygen-rich blood from reaching that area of heart muscle and causes it to die. Without quick treatment, a heart attack can lead to serious problems and even death.

Over time, heart disease can also weaken the heart muscle and lead to heart failure and arrhythmias. Heart failure is a condition in which your heart can't pump enough blood throughout your body. Arrhythmias are problems with the speed or rhythm of your heartbeat. Heart failure is discussed in chapter 3, and arrhythmias are covered in chapter 4.

Other Names for Coronary Artery Disease

- Atherosclerosis
- Coronary heart disease
- Hardening of the arteries
- Heart disease
- Ischemic heart disease
- Narrowing of the arteries

Ischemic Heart Disease

Ischemic heart disease is often referred to as coronary artery disease, abbreviated as CAD. It is a condition in which plaque builds up inside the coronary arteries. These arteries supply your heart muscle with oxygen-rich blood.

Plaque is made up of fat, cholesterol, calcium, and other substances found in the blood. When plaque builds up in the arteries, the condition is called atherosclerosis.

Plaque narrows the arteries and reduces blood flow to your heart muscle. It also makes it more likely that blood clots will form in your arteries. Blood clots can partially or completely block blood flow. Whatever the cause, when the heart muscle does not get enough blood flow, it is known as ischemia.

Ischemic heart disease is the most common type of heart disease. It's the leading cause of death in the United States for both men and women. Other names for ischemic heart disease include atherosclerosis, coronary artery disease, coronary heart disease, hardening of the arteries, heart disease, and narrowing of the arteries.

Causes of Ischemic Heart Disease

Research suggests heart disease starts when certain factors—such as smoking, high amounts of specific fats, high blood pressure, and high amounts of sugar in the blood—damage the inner layers of the coronary arteries. When damage occurs, your body starts a healing process. Excess fatty tissues release compounds that pro-mote this process; however, the body's method of healing causes plaque to build up where the arteries are damaged.

The buildup of plaque in the coronary arteries may start in child-hood. Over time, plaque can narrow or completely block some of your coronary arteries, which reduces the flow of oxygen-rich blood to your heart muscle.

Plaque also can crack, which causes blood cells called platelets to clump together and form blood clots at the site of the cracks. This narrows the arteries more and worsens angina or causes a heart attack.

Risk Factors

Certain traits, conditions, or habits may raise your chance of devel-oping ischemic heart disease. These conditions are known as risk factors. You can control most risk factors and help prevent or delay ischemic heart disease. Other risk factors can't be controlled.

There are many factors that raise the risk of developing ischemic heart disease. The more risk factors you have, the greater your chance of developing ischemic heart disease. Here are some com-mon risk factors for ischemic heart disease:

- **Unhealthy blood cholesterol levels:** This includes high LDL (low-density lipoprotein) cholesterol, sometimes called bad cholesterol, and low HDL (high-density lipo-protein) cholesterol, sometimes called good cholesterol.

- **High blood pressure:** Blood pressure is considered high if it stays at or above 140/90 mmHg (millimeters of mer-cury) over a period of time.

- **Smoking:** This habit can damage and tighten blood ves-sels, raise cholesterol levels, and raise blood pressure. Smoking also doesn't allow enough oxygen to reach the body's tissues.

- **Insulin resistance:** This condition occurs when the body can't use its own insulin properly. Insulin is a hormone that helps move blood sugar into cells where it's used.

- **Diabetes:** This is a disease in which the body's blood sugar level is high because the body doesn't make enough insulin or doesn't use its insulin properly.

- **Overweight or obesity:** Overweight is having extra body weight from muscle, bone, fat, and/or water. Obesity is having a high amount of extra body fat.

- **The metabolic syndrome:** The metabolic syndrome is the name for a group of risk factors linked to overweight and obesity that raise your chance for ischemic heart disease and other health problems, such as diabetes and stroke.

- **Lack of physical activity:** Lack of activity can worsen other risk factors for ischemic heart disease.

- **Age:** As you get older, your risk for ischemic heart disease increases. Genetic or lifestyle factors cause plaque to build up in your arteries as you age. By the time you're middle-aged or older, enough plaque has built up to cause signs or symptoms. In men, the risk for ischemic heart disease increases after age 45. In women, the risk for ischemic heart disease risk increases after age 55.

- **Family history of early heart disease:** Your risk increases if your father or a brother was diagnosed with ischemic heart disease before 55 years of age or if your mother or a sister was diagnosed with ischemic heart disease before 65 years of age.

Although age and a family history of early ischemic heart disease are risk factors, you will not necessarily develop heart disease if you have one or both. Making lifestyle changes and/or taking medicines to treat other risk factors can often lessen genetic influences and prevent heart disease from developing, even in older adults.

Scientists continue to study other possible risk factors for ischemic heart disease. High levels of a protein called C-reactive protein (CRP) in the blood may raise the risk for heart disease and heart attack. High levels of CRP are proof of inflammation in the body. Inflammation is the body's response to injury or infection. Damage to the arteries' inner walls seems to trigger inflammation and help plaque grow. Research is underway to find out whether reducing inflammation, reflected by lowering CRP levels, also can reduce the risk of developing ischemic heart disease and having a heart attack.

High levels of fats called triglycerides in the blood also may raise the risk of ischemic heart disease, particularly in women.

Hormonal Products and Heart Risks

Some women have questions about whether birth control pills, the birth control patch, or the use of menopausal hormone therapy increases their risk for heart disease.

Taking birth control pills or using the patch is generally safe for young, healthy women if they do not smoke. But birth control pills and the patch can pose heart disease risks for some women, especially women older than 35; women with high blood pressure, diabetes, or high cholesterol; and women who smoke.

Additionally, recent studies show women who use the patch may be exposed to more estrogen than women who use the birth control pill. Estrogen is the female hormone in birth control pills and the patch that keeps you from getting pregnant. Research is underway to see if the risk for blood clots, which can lead to heart attack or stroke, is higher in patch users.

Furthermore, for some women, taking menopausal hormone therapy can increase the chances of having a heart attack or stroke; therefore, many doctors recommend patients use hormone therapy at the lowest dose that helps for the shortest time needed. Talk with your doctor if you have questions about these hormonal medications.

Other Factors That Affect Ischemic Heart Disease

Factors such as sleep apnea, stress, and alcohol may also contribute to heart disease:

- **Sleep apnea:** Sleep apnea is a disorder in which your breathing stops or gets very shallow while you're sleeping. Untreated sleep apnea can raise your chances of having high blood pressure, diabetes, and even a heart attack or stroke.

- **Stress:** Research shows that the most commonly reported trigger for a heart attack is an emotionally upsetting event—particularly one involving anger.

- **Alcohol:** Heavy drinking can damage the heart muscle and worsen other risk factors for heart disease. Men should have no more than two drinks containing alcohol a day. Women should have no more than one drink containing alcohol a day.

Signs and Symptoms of Ischemic Heart Disease

Many people who have ischemic heart disease have no signs or symptoms. This is called silent coronary artery disease. It may be present for many years and not diagnosed until a person develops angina, a heart attack, heart failure, or an arrhythmia (an irregular heartbeat).

The severity of symptoms related to ischemic heart disease varies. The symptoms may get more severe as the buildup of plaque continues to narrow the coronary arteries.

Angina

Sometimes, the heart muscle's demand exceeds the available blood supply, and it becomes starved for oxygen. The symptoms that result are called angina.

Angina may take a number of forms and can be quite different from one person to another. However, the most common form of angina is chest pain. The pain and discomfort are often described as pressure, squeezing, burning, or tightness in the chest. The pain or discomfort usually starts in the chest behind the breastbone.

Pain from angina is not always in the chest and may be felt in more than one location at once. It also can occur in the arms, shoulders, neck, jaw, throat, or back. The pain may feel like indigestion. Some people say angina pain is hard to describe or they can't tell exactly where the pain is coming from. Women are more likely to feel discomfort in the neck, jaw, throat, abdomen, or back. Pain from angina is frequently accompanied by other symptoms, such as nausea, shortness of breath, and sweating.

In addition, angina can occur without any pain at all. Sometimes, shortness of breath, sweating, light-headedness, weakness, or nausea may be the only symptom of angina. Shortness of breath without pain is more common in older people and those with diabetes. In elderly people, signs and symptoms of angina may be masked by weakness, dizziness, and confusion. When angina occurs without pain, it is sometimes referred to as an "anginal equivalent."

While all angina is due to inadequate blood flow to the heart muscle, it may occur under different circumstances. In stable angina, the pain or discomfort occurs when the heart must work harder, usually during physical exertion. The episodes of pain tend to be alike and usually last only a short time (five minutes or less). In unstable angina, the pain typically comes as a surprise—often during rest, while sleeping, or with little physical exertion—and the episodes tend to be more severe and last longer (up to 30 minutes). These, and other types of angina, are discussed in greater detail in chapter 38, "Managing Angina."

Because angina has so many possible symptoms and causes, all chest pain should be checked by a doctor. Chest pain that lasts longer than a few minutes and isn't relieved by rest or angina medicine may be a sign of a heart attack. Call 911 right away.

Heart Attack

A heart attack, as mentioned at the beginning of this chapter, occurs when blood flow to a section of heart muscle becomes blocked. You may hear other names for a heart attack, including myocardial infarction (MI), acute myocardial infarction (AMI), acute coronary syndrome, coronary thrombosis, and coronary occlusion.

Heart attack is a leading killer of both men and women in the United States. But today, fortunately, there are excellent treatments that can save lives and prevent disabilities. Treatment is most effective when started within one hour of the beginning of symptoms. If you think you or someone you're with is having a heart attack, call 911 right away.

Each year, about 1.1 million people in the United States have heart attacks, and almost half of them die. Ischemic heart disease—which often results in a heart attack—is the leading killer of both men and women in the United States.

Many more people could recover from heart attacks if they got help faster. Of the people who die from heart attacks, about half die within an hour of the first symptoms and before they reach a hospital.

Other Names for a Heart Attack

- Myocardial infarction or MI
- Acute myocardial infarction or AMI
- Acute coronary syndrome
- Coronary thrombosis
- Coronary occlusion

Causes of a Heart Attack

Most heart attacks occur as a result of ischemic heart disease, the buildup over time of a material called plaque on the inner walls of the coronary arteries. Eventually, a section of plaque can break open, causing a blood clot to form at the site. A heart attack occurs if the clot becomes large enough to cut off most or all of the blood flow through the artery.

The blocked blood flow prevents oxygen-rich blood from reaching the part of the heart muscle fed by the artery. This lack of oxygen damages the heart muscle. If the blockage isn't treated quickly, the damaged heart muscle begins to die.

Heart attacks also can occur due to problems with the very small, microscopic blood vessels of the heart. This condition is called microvascular disease. It's believed to be more common in women than in men.

Another less common cause of heart attack is a severe spasm (tightening) of a coronary artery, which cuts off blood flow through the artery. These spasms can occur in coronary arteries that don't have heart disease. It's not always clear what causes a coronary artery spasm, but sometimes it can be related to taking certain drugs, such as cocaine; emotional stress or pain; exposure to extreme cold; or cigarette smoking.

Act Fast for Heart Attack Symptoms

Sometimes the signs and symptoms of a heart attack happen suddenly, but they can also develop slowly—over hours, days, and even weeks—before a heart attack occurs.

Acting fast at the first sign of heart attack symptoms can save your life and limit damage to your heart. Treatment is most effective when started within one hour of the beginning of symptoms. The sooner you get emergency help, the less damage there will be to your heart.

If you think you or someone you know may be having a heart attack:

- Call 911 within a few minutes—five at the most—of the start of symptoms.
- If your symptoms stop completely in less than five minutes, still call your doctor.
- Only take an ambulance to the hospital. Going in a private car can delay treatment. Don't drive yourself or anyone else to the hospital.
- Take a nitroglycerin pill if your doctor has prescribed it.

Signs and Symptoms of Heart Attack

Not all heart attacks begin with the sudden, crushing pain often shown on TV or in the movies. The warning signs and symptoms of a heart attack aren't the same for everyone. Many heart attacks start slowly as mild pain or discomfort. Some people don't have symptoms at all (called a silent heart attack).

The most common symptom of heart attack is chest pain or discomfort. Most heart attacks involve discomfort in the center of the chest lasting for more than a few minutes or intermittently. The discomfort can feel like uncomfortable pressure, squeezing, fullness, or pain. It can be mild or severe. Heart attack pain can sometimes feel like indigestion or heartburn.

The symptoms of angina can be similar to the symptoms of a heart attack. Angina that doesn't go away or that changes from its usual pattern (occurs more frequently or at rest) can signal the beginning of a heart attack and should be checked by a doctor right away.

Other common signs and symptoms a person can have during a heart attack include the following: upper body discomfort in one or both arms or the back, neck, jaw, or stomach; shortness of breath, often occurring with or before chest discomfort; nausea (feeling sick to your stomach), vomiting, light-headedness or fainting, or breaking out in a cold sweat

Not everyone having a heart attack experiences the typical symptoms. If you've already had a heart attack, your symptoms may not be the same for another one. The more signs and symptoms you have, the more likely it is you're having a heart attack.

Excerpted and adapted from "Coronary Artery Disease," February 2009, "Angina," March 2010, and "Heart Attack," March 2008, all three produced by the National Heart, Lung, and Blood Institute (NHLBI, www.nhlbi.nih.gov). Additional information about birth control pills and menopausal hormone therapy excerpted and adapted from "Frequently Asked Questions about Heart Disease," Office on Women's Health (www.womenshealth.gov), February 2, 2009.

Chapter 3

Heart Failure and Cardiomyopathy

Heart failure is a condition in which the heart can't pump enough blood to meet the body's needs. In some cases, the heart can't fill with enough blood. In other cases, the heart can't pump blood to the rest of the body with enough force. Some people have both problems.

The term heart failure doesn't mean your heart has stopped or is about to stop working. However, heart failure is a serious condition that requires medical care.

While heart failure has many different underlying causes, it can be divided into two basic categories. Systolic heart failure occurs when the heart muscle is weak or damaged and cannot pump force-fully during systole, the squeezing phase of the heart cycle. This is most often the result of ischemic heart disease or cardiomyopathy, which are discussed in the following sections.

Diastolic heart failure occurs when the heart cannot properly fill with blood during diastole, the period between heartbeats. If the heart chambers do not fill well, less blood will be pumped when the heart beats. The most common cause of diastolic heart failure—also called diastolic dysfunction—is abnormal stiffness of the heart muscle. The muscle cannot relax properly to allow normal blood filling. High blood pressure, ischemic heart disease, diabetes, and aging are the most common reasons for stiffness to develop.

Although people often think of heart failure as a disease caused by a weak heart muscle, diastolic heart failure is actually more common than systolic heart failure. Symptoms of heart failure are the same in most cases whether it is due to systolic or diastolic dysfunction.

Symptoms of heart failure, sometimes called dropsy, develop when the heart is not moving blood effectively. The condition can affect the right side of the heart only, or it can affect both sides of the heart. Most cases involve both sides of the heart.

Right-side heart failure occurs if the heart can't pump enough blood to the lungs to pick up oxygen. Left-side heart failure occurs if the heart can't pump enough oxygen-rich blood to the rest of the body.

Right-side heart failure may cause fluid to build up in the feet, ankles, legs, liver, abdomen, and the veins in the neck. Right-side and left-side heart failure also may cause shortness of breath and fatigue.

Heart failure is a very common condition. Both children and adults can have heart failure, although the symptoms and treatments differ.

Currently, heart failure has no cure. However, treatments—such as medicines and lifestyle changes—can help people live longer and more active lives. Researchers continue to study new ways to treat heart failure and its complications.

Causes of Heart Failure

Conditions that damage, overwork, or stiffen the heart muscle can cause heart failure. The heart isn't able to fill with or pump blood as well as it should.

As the blood circulated by the heart drops, certain proteins and other substances may be released into the blood. These substances have a toxic effect on the heart and blood flow, and they worsen heart failure.

The most common causes of heart failure are ischemic heart disease, high blood pressure, and diabetes. Treating these problems can prevent or improve heart failure.

Ischemic Heart Disease

Ischemic heart disease was discussed in chapter 2. To summarize, it is a condition in which a substance called plaque builds up inside the coronary arteries. These arteries supply oxygen-rich blood to your heart muscle. When blood flow to the heart is blocked, it can lead to chest pain or discomfort called angina, a heart attack, heart damage, or even death. Ischemic heart disease can cause systolic heart failure, by weakening the heart muscle, or diastolic heart failure, by making the heart muscle abnormally stiff.

High Blood Pressure

Blood pressure is the force of blood pushing against the walls of the arteries. If this pressure rises and stays high over time, it can weaken your heart and lead to plaque buildup. When blood pressure is high for long periods of time, the heart muscle will often thicken in response, which increases its stiffness. Blood pressure is considered high if it stays at or above 140/90 mmHg over time. The "mmHg" stands for millimeters of mercury— the units used to measure blood pressure. If you have diabetes or chronic kidney disease, high blood pressure is defined as 130/80 mmHg or higher.

Diabetes

Diabetes is a disease in which the body's blood glucose, or blood sugar, level is too high. Normally, the body breaks down food into glucose and then carries it to cells throughout the body. The cells use a hormone called insulin to turn the glucose into energy. In diabetes, the body doesn't make enough insulin or doesn't use its insulin properly. Over time, high blood sugar levels can damage and weaken the heart muscle and the blood vessels around the heart, leading to heart failure. Abnormal stiffness of the heart is also common in people with diabetes.

Other Causes

Other diseases and conditions also can lead to heart failure, such as the following:

- **Cardiomyopathy:** Cardiomyopathy, also called heart muscle disease, is discussed in detail later in this chapter.

- **Arrhythmias, or irregular heartbeats:** These heart problems may be present at birth or due to heart disease or heart defects. Chapter 4 provides more information about arrhythmias.

- **Heart valve disease:** Problems with the heart valves may be present at birth or due to infection, heart attack, or damage from heart disease. See chapter 5, "Heart Murmurs and Structural Heart Disease," for more information.

- **Congenital heart defects:** These heart problems are present at birth. They are also discussed in chapter 5.

Other factors also can injure the heart muscle and lead to heart failure. Examples include treatments for cancer (such as radiation and chemotherapy), thyroid disorders (having either too much or too little thyroid hormone in the body), alcohol abuse, the abuse of cocaine and other illegal drugs, human immunodeficiency virus/acquired immunodeficiency syndrome (HIV/AIDS), and too much vitamin E. Heart damage from obstructive sleep apnea may also cause heart failure to worsen, and treating this sleep problem may improve heart failure.

Risk Factors for Heart Failure

About 5.7 million people in the United States have heart failure, and it results in about 300,000 deaths each year. The number of people who have heart failure is growing.

Heart failure is more common in the following groups:

- **People who are 65 years old or older:** Aging can weaken the heart muscle and cause increased stiffness. Older people also may have had long-term diseases which have caused heart failure. Heart failure is the most common reason for hospital visits among people on Medicare.

- **African Americans:** African Americans are more likely than people of other races to have heart failure. They're also more likely to have symptoms at a younger age, have more hospital visits due to heart failure, and die from heart failure.

- **People who are overweight:** Excess weight puts strain on the heart. Being overweight also increases your risk of heart disease and type 2 diabetes. These diseases can lead to heart failure.

Additionally, men have a higher rate of heart failure than women.

Children who have congenital heart defects also can develop heart failure. These defects occur if the heart, heart valves, or blood vessels near the heart don't form correctly while a baby is in the womb. Congenital heart defects can make the heart work harder and weaken the heart muscle, leading to heart failure.

Signs and Symptoms of Heart Failure

The most common signs and symptoms of heart failure are shortness of breath or trouble breathing, fatigue, and swelling in the ankles, feet, legs, abdomen, and veins in the neck. All these symptoms are the result of inadequate blood circulation and fluid buildup in your body. When symptoms start, you may feel tired and short of breath after routine physical effort, like climbing stairs.

As your heart failure worsens, symptoms get worse. You may begin to feel tired and short of breath after getting dressed or walking across the room. Some people have shortness of breath while lying flat.

Fluid buildup from heart failure also causes weight gain, frequent urination, and a cough that's worse at night and when you're lying down. This cough may be a sign of acute pulmonary edema, a condition in which too much fluid builds up in your lungs. Acute pulmonary edema requires emergency treatment.

Cardiomyopathy

Cardiomyopathy, a cause of heart failure, refers to diseases of the heart muscle. These diseases have a variety of causes, symptoms, and treatments.

The most common form of cardiomyopathy is ischemic cardiomyopathy. In ischemic cardiomyopathy, problems stem from poor blood flow through the heart muscle or from a prior heart attack. However, not all cardiomyopathy is due to ischemia. Cardiomyopathy due to other diseases is called nonischemic cardiomyopathy. In nonischemic cardiomyopathy, the heart muscle becomes enlarged, thick, or rigid. In rare cases, the muscle tissue in the heart is replaced with scar tissue.

As cardiomyopathy worsens, the heart becomes weaker. It's less able to pump blood through the body and maintain a normal electrical rhythm, which can lead to heart failure or arrhythmia. This weakening of the heart also can cause other severe complications, such as heart valve problems.

Cardiomyopathy can be acquired or inherited. Acquired means you aren't born with the disease, but you develop it due to another disease, condition, or factor. Inherited means your parents passed the gene for the disease on to you. Researchers continue to look for the genetic links to cardiomyopathy. They also continue to explore how these links cause or contribute to the various types of cardiomyopathy. Many times, the cause of cardiomyopathy isn't known. This is often the case when the disease occurs in children.

Some people who have cardiomyopathy have no signs or symptoms and need no treatment. For other people, the disease develops rapidly, symptoms are severe, and serious complications occur.

Treatments for cardiomyopathy include lifestyle changes, medicines, surgery, implanted devices to correct arrhythmias, and a nonsurgical procedure. These treatments can control symptoms, reduce complications, and stop the disease from getting worse.

There are several different types of cardiomyopathy described in the following sections. Within each type, individual kinds of cardiomyopathy are often named according to the underlying cause (for example, diabetic cardiomyopathy, asymmetric septal hypertrophy, or right ventricular cardiomyopathy).

Dilated Cardiomyopathy

Dilated cardiomyopathy is the most common type. It mostly occurs in adults aged 20 to 60. Men are more likely than women to have this type of cardiomyopathy.

Dilated cardiomyopathy affects the heart's ventricles and atria—the lower and upper chambers of the heart, respectively. The disease often starts in the left ventricle, the heart's main pumping chamber. The heart muscle begins to dilate (stretch and become thinner). This causes the inside of the chamber to enlarge. The problem often spreads to the right ventricle and then to the atria as the disease gets worse.

When the chambers dilate, the heart muscle doesn't contract normally. Also, the heart can't pump blood very well. Over time, the heart becomes weaker and heart failure can occur. Dilated cardiomyopathy also can lead to heart valve problems, arrhythmias, and blood clots in the heart.

Most dilated cardiomyopathy is related to ischemic heart disease. For nonischemic dilated cardiomyopathy, the cause is not known in more than half of the cases. As many as one-third of the people who have nonischemic dilated cardiomyopathy inherit it from their parents. Certain diseases, conditions, and substances also can cause the disease, such as the following:

- Thyroid disease, viral hepatitis, and HIV

- Infections, especially viral infections that inflame the heart muscle

- Alcohol, especially if you also have a poor diet

- Complications during the last month of pregnancy or within five months of birth

- Certain toxins, such as cobalt

- Certain drugs (such as cocaine and amphetamines) and two medicines used to treat cancer (doxorubicin and daunorubicin)

Hypertrophic Cardiomyopathy

Hypertrophic cardiomyopathy is very common and can affect people of any age. About one out of every 500 people has this type of cardiomyopathy. It affects men and women equally. Hypertrophic cardiomyopathy is the most common cause of sudden cardiac arrest (SCA) in young people, including young athletes.

Despite similar names, hypertrophic cardiomyopathy is not the same thing as hypertensive heart disease. Both involve thickening of the heart muscle, but they occur for different reasons. In hypertensive heart disease, thickening is a result of excessive stress on the heart from high blood pressure. Hypertrophic cardiomyopathy is a genetic disease, and it frequently occurs in people with no other medical problems.

Hypertrophic cardiomyopathy is due to a mutation (change) in one or more genes important in heart muscle. More than one kind of mutation can cause the disorder, and this may explain why the symptoms and severity of hypertrophic cardiomyopathy can vary from person to person.

Most people with hypertrophic cardiomyopathy have a family history of the disorder. However, hypertrophic cardiomyopathy can affect people who do not have any affected family members.

The key sign of hypertrophic cardiomyopathy is abnormal thickening of the walls of the ventricles. This can affect the entire heart or just parts of it. When it affects only one portion of the heart, it is often called asymmetric hypertrophic cardiomyopathy. The thickening can be quite extreme, and the walls can be several times normal width. Despite this thickening, the ventricle size is often normal or smaller than normal because the growth is in the walls of the heart, rather than the internal spaces.

Depending on its location in the heart and its severity, hypertrophic cardiomyopathy may block blood flow out of the ventricle. When this happens, the condition is called obstructive hypertrophic cardiomyopathy. In some cases, the septum thickens and bulges into the left ventricle. (The septum is the wall that divides the left and right sides of the heart.) In both cases, blood flow out of the left ventricle is blocked.

As a result of the blockage, the ventricle must work much harder to pump blood out to the body. Symptoms can include chest pain, dizziness, shortness of breath, or fainting.

Changes in the shape of the heart from hypertrophic cardiomyopathy can also affect the heart's mitral valve, causing blood to leak backward through the valve. This can lead to impaired heart function.

Whether or not obstruction occurs, the thickened muscle may make the inside of the left ventricle smaller, so it holds less blood. The walls of the ventricle also may stiffen. As a result, the ventricle is less able to relax and fill with blood. This may lead to heart failure due to diastolic dysfunction. Symptoms may include an inability to exercise or extreme fatigue with little physical activity. However, some people who have hypertrophic cardiomyopathy have no signs or symptoms, and the condition doesn't affect their lives.

Thickening of the heart muscle is not the only problem in hypertrophic cardiomyopathy. The affected heart muscle is also electrically abnormal and prone to developing arrhythmias, which are electrical short-circuits in the heart. Arrhythmias are discussed in greater detail in chapter 4. Arrhythmias do not develop in everyone with hypertrophic cardiomyopathy. However, they are common, and tend to occur during vigorous exercise. Severity can range from mild to fatal.

Sometimes, arrhythmias are the clues that lead to a diagnosis of hypertrophic cardiomyopathy. Unfortunately, sudden cardiac death is sometimes the first symptom. When teenage athletes die suddenly during sports events, they are often found to have had undiagnosed hypertrophic cardiomyopathy.

If you have hypertrophic cardiomyopathy, talk to your doctor about what types and amounts of physical activity are safe for you. Some people with hypertrophic cardiomyopathy have an implantable cardiac defibrillator (ICD) placed as a precautionary measure. ICD's are discussed in more detail in chapter 24.

Restrictive Cardiomyopathy

Restrictive cardiomyopathy tends to mostly affect older adults. In this type of the disease, the ventricles become stiff and rigid due to abnormal tissue, such as scar tissue, replacing the normal heart muscle.

As a result, the ventricles can't relax normally and fill with blood, and the atria become enlarged. Over time, blood flow in the heart is reduced. This can lead to problems such as heart failure or arrhythmias.

Certain diseases and conditions can cause restrictive cardiomyopathy, including the following:

- **Hemochromatosis:** This is a disease in which too much iron builds up in your body. The extra iron is toxic to the body and can damage the organs, including the heart.

- **Sarcoidosis:** This is a disease that causes inflammation (swelling). It can affect various organs in the body. The swelling is due to an abnormal immune response. This abnormal response causes tiny lumps of cells to form in the body's organs, including the heart.

- **Amyloidosis:** This is a disease in which abnormal proteins build up in the body's organs, including the heart.

- **Connective tissue disorders:** These are disorders where the body's immune system attacks normal organs, such as lupus and scleroderma.

Arrhythmogenic Right Ventricular Dysplasia

Arrhythmogenic right ventricular dysplasia (ARVD) is a rare type of cardiomyopathy. ARVD occurs when the muscle tissue in the right ventricle dies and is replaced with scar tissue.

This process disrupts the heart's electrical signals and causes arrhythmias. Symptoms include palpitations and fainting after physical activity.

ARVD usually affects teens or young adults. It can cause SCA in young athletes. Fortunately, such deaths are rare.

Researchers think arrhythmogenic right ventricular dysplasia is an inherited disease.

Excerpted and adapted from "Heart Failure," January 2010, and "Cardiomyopathy," December 2008, both produced by the National Heart, Lung, and Blood Institute (NHLBI, www.nhlbi.nih.gov), with supplemental information added by David A. Cooke, MD, FACP, May 2010.

Chapter 4

Arrhythmias and Electrical Heart Disease

An arrhythmia is a problem with the rate or rhythm of the heartbeat. During an arrhythmia, the heart can beat too fast, too slow, or with an irregular rhythm.

A heartbeat that is too fast is called tachycardia. A heartbeat that is too slow is called bradycardia.

Most arrhythmias, also called dysrhythmias, are harmless, but some can be serious or even life threatening. When the heart rate is too fast, too slow, or irregular, the heart may not be able to pump enough blood to the body. Lack of blood flow can damage the brain, heart, and other organs.

Many arrhythmias cause no signs or symptoms. When signs or symptoms are present, the most common include palpitations (feeling your heart is skipping a beat, fluttering, or beating too hard or fast), a slow heartbeat, an irregular heartbeat, and pauses between heartbeats. More serious signs and symptoms include anxiety; weakness, dizziness, and light-headedness;

fainting or nearly fainting; sweating; shortness of breath; and chest pain.

To understand arrhythmias, it helps to understand the heart's internal electrical system because the heart's electrical system controls the rate and rhythm of the heartbeat. (For more information about how the heart's electrical system works, see chapter 1, "How the Heart and Circulatory System Work.") A problem with any part of the heartbeat process can cause an arrhythmia. For example, in atrial fibrillation, electrical signals travel through the atria in a fast and disorganized way. This causes the atria to quiver instead of contract.

There are many types of arrhythmia, and the four main types are premature (extra) beats, supraventricular arrhythmias, ventricular arrhythmias, and bradyarrhythmias. The outlook for a person with an arrhythmia depends on the type and severity of the arrhythmia. Even serious arrhythmias often can be successfully treated. Most people who have arrhythmias are able to live normal, healthy lives.

Premature Beats

Premature (extra) beats are the most common type of arrhythmia. They're harmless most of the time and often don't cause any symptoms.

When symptoms do occur, they usually feel like fluttering in the chest or a feeling of a skipped beat. Most of the time, premature beats need no treatment, especially in healthy people.

Premature beats that occur in the atria are called premature atrial contractions, or PACs. Premature beats that occur in the ventricles are called premature ventricular contractions, or PVCs.

In most cases, premature beats occur naturally rather than due to any heart disease. But certain heart diseases can cause premature beats. Premature beats also can happen because of stress, too much exercise, or too much caffeine or nicotine.

Supraventricular Arrhythmias

Supraventricular arrhythmias are tachycardias (fast heart rates) that start in the atria or the atrioventricular (AV) node. The AV node is a group of cells located between the atria and the ventricles.

Types of supraventricular arrhythmias include atrial fibrillation, atrial flutter, paroxysmal supraventricular tachycardia, and Wolff-Parkinson-White syndrome.

Atrial Fibrillation

Atrial fibrillation (also called AF) is a very fast and irregular contraction of the atria. It the most common type of serious arrhythmia, and because of its significance, it is discussed in greater detail later in this chapter.

Atrial Flutter

Atrial flutter is similar to AF, but instead of the electrical signals spreading through the atria in a fast and irregular rhythm, they travel in a fast and regular rhythm. Atrial flutter is much less common than AF, but it has similar symptoms and complications.

Paroxysmal Supraventricular Tachycardia

Paroxysmal supraventricular tachycardia is abbreviated PSVT. It is a very fast heart rate that begins and ends suddenly. PSVT occurs due to problems with the electrical connection between the atria and the ventricles.

In PSVT, electrical signals that begin in the atria and travel to the ventricles can reenter the atria, causing extra heartbeats. This type of arrhythmia usually isn't dangerous and tends to occur in young people. It can happen during vigorous exercise.

A special type of PSVT is called Wolff-Parkinson-White (WPW) syndrome. WPW syndrome is a condition in which the heart's electrical signals travel along an extra pathway from the atria to the ventricles. This extra pathway disrupts the timing of the heart's electrical signals and can cause the ventricles to beat very fast, which can be life threatening.

Ventricular Arrhythmias

These arrhythmias start in the ventricles. They can be very dangerous and usually require medical attention right away.

Ventricular arrhythmias include ventricular tachycardia and ventricular fibrillation (v-fib). Coronary heart disease, heart attack, weakened heart muscle, and other problems can cause ventricular arrhythmias.

Ventricular Tachycardia

Ventricular tachycardia is a fast, regular beating of the ventricles that may last for only a few seconds or for much longer. A few beats of ventricular tachycardia often don't cause problems. However, episodes that last for more than a few seconds can be dangerous. The heart can beat so rapidly that it is unable to move blood effectively. Ventricular tachycardia can turn into other, more dangerous arrhythmias, such as v-fib.

Ventricular Fibrillation

V-fib occurs when disorganized electrical signals make the ventricles quiver instead of pump normally. Without the ventricles pumping blood out to the body, you'll lose consciousness within seconds and die within minutes if not treated. To prevent death, the condition must be treated right away with an electric shock to the heart called defibrillation.

V-fib may happen during or after a heart attack or in someone whose heart is already weak because of another condition. Health experts think most of the sudden cardiac deaths that occur every year (about 335,000) are due to v-fib.

Torsades de pointes (torsades) is a type of v-fib that causes a unique pattern on an EKG. Certain medicines or imbalanced amounts of potassium, calcium, or magnesium in the bloodstream can cause this condition. People who have long QT syndrome are at higher risk for torsades. People who have this condition need to be careful about taking certain antibiotics, heart medicines, and over-the-counter medicines that alter electrical activity in the heart.

Long QT Syndrome

Long QT syndrome is a disorder of the heart's electrical activity. It may cause you to develop a sudden, uncontrollable, and dangerous arrhythmia in response to exercise or stress.

The term "long QT" refers to an abnormal pattern seen on an EKG. The QT interval, recorded on the EKG, corresponds to the time during which the lower chambers of your heart are triggered to contract and then build the potential to contract again.

Normally the QT interval of the heartbeat lasts about a third of each heartbeat cycle on the EKG. However, in people who have long QT syndrome, the QT interval usually lasts longer than normal. This can upset the careful timing of the heartbeat and trigger a dangerous, abnormal rhythm.

Bradyarrhythmias

Bradyarrhythmias are arrhythmias in which the heart rate is slower than normal. If the heart rate is too slow, not enough blood reaches the brain, which can cause you to lose consciousness.

In adults, a heart rate slower than 60 beats per minute is considered a bradyarrhythmia. Some people normally have slow heart rates, especially those who are very physically fit. For them, a heartbeat slower than 60 beats per minute isn't dangerous and doesn't cause symptoms. But in other people, bradyarrhythmia can be a symptom of a serious disease or other condition.

Bradyarrhythmias can be caused by heart attacks or conditions that harm or change the heart's electrical activity, such as an underactive thyroid gland or aging. An imbalance of chemicals or other substances, such as potassium, in the blood can lead to bradyarrhythmias, and so can some medicines, such as beta blockers.

Bradyarrhythmias also can occur as a result of severe bundle branch block. Bundle branch block is a condition in which an electrical signal traveling down either or both bundle branches is delayed or blocked.

When this happens, the ventricles don't contract at exactly the same time, as they should. As a result, the heart has to work harder to pump blood to the body. The cause of bundle branch block often is an existing heart condition.

Arrhythmias in Children

A child's heart rate normally decreases as he or she gets older. A newborn's heart beats between 95 to 160 times a minute. A one-year-old's heart beats between 90 to 150 times a minute, and a six- to eight-year-old's heart beats between 60 to 110 times a minute.

A baby or child's heart can beat faster or slower than normal for many reasons. Like adults, when children are active, their hearts will beat faster. When they're sleeping, their hearts will beat slower. Their heart rates can speed up and slow down as they breathe in and out. All these changes are normal.

Some children are born with heart defects that cause arrhythmias. In other children, arrhythmias can develop later in childhood.

Causes of Arrhythmia

An arrhythmia can occur if the electrical signals that control the heartbeat are delayed or blocked. This can happen if the special nerve cells that produce electrical signals don't work properly or if electrical signals don't travel normally through the heart.

An arrhythmia also can occur if another part of the heart starts to produce electrical signals. This adds to the signals from the special nerve cells and disrupts the normal heartbeat. This may occur when there is damage or disease of the heart muscle, such as in hypertrophic cardiomyopathy.

Smoking, heavy alcohol use, use of certain drugs (such as cocaine or amphetamines), use of certain prescription or over-the-counter medicines, or too much caffeine or nicotine can lead to arrhythmias in some people.

Strong emotional stress or anger can make the heart work harder, raise blood pressure, and release stress hormones. In some people, these reactions can lead to arrhythmias.

A heart attack or an underlying condition that damages the heart's electrical system also can cause arrhythmias. Examples of such conditions include high blood pressure, coronary heart disease, heart failure, overactive or underactive thyroid gland (too much or too little thyroid hormone produced), and rheumatic heart disease.

In some arrhythmias, such as Wolff-Parkinson-White syndrome, the underlying heart defect that causes the arrhythmia is congenital. Sometimes, the cause of an arrhythmia can't be found.

Risk Factors for Arrhythmia

Millions of Americans have arrhythmias. They're very common in older adults. Most serious arrhythmias affect people older than 60 because older adults are more likely to have heart disease and other health problems that can lead to arrhythmias. Older adults also tend to be more sensitive to the side effects of medicines, some of which can cause arrhythmias. Some medicines used to treat arrhythmias can even cause arrhythmias as a side effect.

Arrhythmias are more common in people who have diseases or conditions that weaken the heart, such as the following:

- Heart attack
- Heart failure or cardiomyopathy, which weakens the heart and changes the way electrical signals move around the heart
- Heart tissue that's too thick or stiff or that hasn't formed normally

- Leaking or narrowed heart valves, which make the heart work too hard and can lead to heart failure

- Congenital heart defects (problems that are present at birth) that affect the heart's structure or function

- High blood pressure

- Infections that damage the heart muscle or the sac around the heart

- Diabetes, which increases the risk of high blood pressure and coronary heart disease

- Sleep apnea (when breathing becomes shallow or stops during sleep), which can stress the heart because the heart doesn't get enough oxygen

- An overactive or underactive thyroid gland (too much or too little thyroid hormone in the body)

Also, several other risk factors can increase risk for arrhythmias. Examples include heart surgery, certain drugs (such as cocaine or amphetamines), or an imbalance of chemicals or other substances (such as potassium) in the bloodstream.

Atrial Fibrillation

As mentioned previously, atrial fibrillation is the most common type of arrhythmia. AF, sometimes referred to as A fib or auricular fibrillation, occurs when rapid, disorganized electrical signals cause the atria, the two upper chambers of the heart, to fibrillate. The term *fibrillate* means to contract very fast and irregularly as a result of damage to the heart's electrical system. The damage most often is the result of other conditions, such as coronary heart disease (also called ischemic heart disease or coronary artery disease) or high blood pressure, that affect the health of the heart, but sometimes the cause of AF is unknown.

In AF, blood pools in the atria and isn't pumped completely into the ventricles, the heart's two lower chambers. As a result, the heart's upper and lower chambers don't work together as they should.

There are sometimes signs and symptoms of atrial fibrillation. These include palpitations (feeling your heart is skipping a beat, fluttering, or beating too hard or fast), shortness of breath, weakness or difficulty exercising, chest pain, dizziness or fainting, fatigue, and confusion. Often people who have AF may not feel symptoms. However, even when not noticed, AF can increase the risk of stroke. In some people, AF can cause chest pain or heart failure, particularly when the heart rhythm is very rapid.

AF may occur rarely or every now and then, or it may become a persistent or permanent heart rhythm lasting for years.

Understanding the Electrical Problem in Atrial Fibrillation

In AF, the heart's electrical signals don't begin in the SA (sino-atrial) node. Instead, they begin in another part of the atria or in the nearby pulmonary veins. The signals don't travel normally, and they may spread throughout the atria in a rapid, disorganized way. This can cause the atria to fibrillate.

The abnormal electrical signals flood the AV node with electrical impulses. As a result, the ventricles also begin to beat very fast. However, the AV node can't conduct the signals to the ventricles as fast as they arrive. So even though the ventricles may be beating faster than normal, they aren't beating as fast as the atria.

Thus, the atria and ventricles no longer beat in a coordinated way. This creates a fast and irregular heart rhythm. In AF, the ventricles may beat 100 to 175 times a minute, in contrast to the normal rate of 60 to 100 beats a minute.

When this happens, blood isn't pumped into the ventricles as well as it should be. Also, the amount of blood pumped out of the ventricles to the body is based on the randomness of the atrial beats.

The body may get rapid, small amounts of blood and occasional larger amounts of blood. The amount depends on how much blood has flowed from the atria to the ventricles with each beat.

Most of the symptoms of AF are related to how fast the heart is beating. If medicines or age slow the heart rate, the symptoms are minimized.

AF may be brief, with symptoms that come and go and end on their own, or the condition may be persistent and require treatment. Sometimes AF is permanent, and medicines or other treatments can't restore a normal heart rhythm.

Types of Atrial Fibrillation

There are several different types of atrial fibrillation:

- **Paroxysmal atrial fibrillation:** In paroxysmal atrial fibrillation, the abnormal electrical signals and rapid heart rate begin suddenly and then stop on their own. Symptoms can be mild or severe and last for seconds, minutes, hours, or days.

- **Persistent atrial fibrillation:** Persistent AF is a condition in which the abnormal heart rhythm continues until it's stopped with treatment.

- **Permanent atrial fibrillation:** Permanent AF is a condition in which a normal heart rhythm can't be restored with the usual treatments. Both paroxysmal and persistent AF may become more frequent and, over time, may result in permanent AF.

Risk Factors for Atrial Fibrillation

More than two million people in the United States have atrial fibrillation. It affects both men and women. The risk of AF increases as you age. This is mostly because as you get older, your risk for heart disease and other conditions that can cause AF also increases.

However, about half of the people who have AF are younger than 75. AF is uncommon in children.

AF is more common in people who have heart diseases or conditions, such as ischemic heart disease (coronary heart disease), heart failure, rheumatic heart disease, structural heart defects (such as mitral valve disorders), hypertension, obesity, pericarditis (a condition in which the membrane, or sac, around your heart is inflamed), or congenital heart defects. It is also more common in people with sick sinus syndrome, a condition in which the heart's electrical signals don't fire properly and the heart rate slows down; sometimes the heart switches back and forth between a slow rate and a fast rate. And AF is more common in people who are having heart attacks or who have just had surgery.

Some conditions other than those directly related to the heart can also increase AF risk. These include hyperthyroidism (too much thyroid hormone), diabetes, and lung disease. Drinking large amounts of alcohol—especially binge drinking—can increase risk. Even modest amounts of alcohol can trigger AF in some people. Caffeine or psychological stress also may trigger AF. The metabolic syndrome, a group of risk factors that increase the risk of heart disease and other health problems, increases your risk of AF. Additionally, some evidence suggests people who have sleep apnea are at greater risk, and recent research suggests people who receive high-dose steroid therapy are at increased risk of AF. This therapy, commonly used for asthma and certain inflammatory conditions, may act as a trigger in people who already have other AF risk factors.

Atrial Fibrillation Complications

AF has two major complications—stroke and heart failure.

During AF, the atria don't pump all their blood to the ventricles, and some blood pools in the atria. When this happens, a blood clot (also called a thrombus) can form. If the clot breaks off and travels to the brain, it can cause a stroke. (A clot that forms in one part of the body and travels in the bloodstream to another part of the body is called an embolus.) Blood-thinning medicines to reduce the risk of stroke are a very important part of treatment for people with AF.

Heart failure occurs when the heart can't pump enough blood to meet the body's needs. AF can lead to heart failure because the ventricles are beating very fast and aren't able to properly fill with blood to pump out to the body.

Heart Block

Heart block is a problem with the heart's electrical system. It occurs when the electrical signal is slowed or disrupted as it moves through the heart. You can be born with heart block (congenital) or you can acquire it.

One form of congenital heart block occurs in the babies of women who have autoimmune diseases such as lupus. People who have these diseases make proteins called antibodies. In pregnant women, these antibodies can cross the placenta (the organ that attaches the umbilical cord to the mother's womb). They can damage the baby's heart and lead to congenital heart block. Congenital heart defects (problems with the heart's structure) also may cause congenital heart block. Often doctors don't know what causes these defects.

Acquired heart block is more common than congenital heart block. A number of factors, such as diseases, surgery, medicines, and other conditions, can cause acquired heart block. The most common cause of acquired heart block is damage to the heart from a heart attack. Other diseases that can cause heart block include ischemic heart disease, myocarditis (inflammation of the heart muscle), heart failure, rheumatic fever, and cardiomyopathy. Other diseases may increase the risk for heart block. These include sarcoidosis and the degenerative muscle disorders, Lev disease and Lenègre disease.

Certain types of surgery also may damage the heart's electrical system and lead to heart block. Exposure to toxic substances and taking certain medicines, including digitalis and beta blockers, also may cause heart block. Doctors closely watch people who are taking these medicines for signs of problems.

In some cases, acquired heart block may go away if the factor causing it is treated or resolved. For example, heart block that occurs after a heart attack or surgery may go away after recovery. Also, if a medicine is causing heart block, the condition may go away if the medicine is stopped or the dosage is lowered. However, you shouldn't change the way you take your medicines unless your doctor tells you to.

The three types of heart block are first degree, second degree, and third degree. First degree is the least severe and third degree is the most severe. This is true for both congenital and acquired heart block.

The symptoms and severity of heart block depend on which type you have. First-degree heart block rarely causes severe symptoms. Second-degree heart block may result in the heart skipping a beat or beats. This type of heart block also can make you feel dizzy or faint. Third-degree heart block limits the heart's ability to pump blood to the rest of the body and may cause fatigue, dizziness, and fainting. These symptoms may point to other health problems as well. If these symptoms are new or severe, call 911 or go to the hospital emergency room. Third-degree heart block requires prompt treatment because it can be fatal. If you have milder symptoms, talk to your doctor right away to find out whether you need prompt treatment.

Pacemakers

A pacemaker is used to treat third-degree heart block and some cases of second-degree heart block. This device uses electrical pulses to make the heart beat at a normal rate. For more information about pacemakers, see chapter 25.

First-Degree Heart Block

In first-degree heart block, the electrical signal is slowed as it moves through the heart. When this occurs between the atria and the ventricles, it appears as a slightly longer, flatter line between the P and the R waves on an electrocardiogram.

First-degree heart block rarely causes any symptoms. Well-trained athletes and young people are at higher risk for first-degree heart block caused by an overly active vagus nerve. Activity in this nerve slows the heart rate. Some medicines, such as digitalis, also may trigger first-degree heart block.

First-degree heart block usually doesn't require treatment.

Second-Degree Heart Block

In this type of heart block, electrical signals between the atria and the ventricles are slowed to a large degree. Some signals can't reach the ventricles. If the signal is blocked before it reaches the ventricles, they won't contract and pump blood to the lungs and the rest of the body.

Second-degree heart block is divided into two different types, Mobitz type I and Mobitz type II. In Mobitz type I (also known as Wenckebach block), the electrical signals are delayed more and more with each heartbeat until the heart skips a beat.

Sometimes people with Mobitz type I feel dizzy or have other symptoms. This type of second-degree heart block is less serious than Mobitz type II.

In Mobitz type II, some of the electrical signals also don't reach the ventricles. However, the pattern is less regular than in Mobitz type I. Some signals move between the atria and the ventricles normally, while others are blocked. Mobitz type II is less common than type I, but it's usually more severe. Some people with type II need pacemakers to maintain their heart rates. Mobitz type II heart block is often a sign that heart block will very soon worsen to third-degree heart block.

Third-Degree Heart Block

In this type of heart block, none of the electrical signals reach the ventricles. This type also is called complete heart block or complete AV block.

When complete heart block occurs, special areas in the ventricles may create electrical signals to cause the ventricles to contract. This natural backup system is slow and isn't coordinated with the contraction of the atria.

Complete heart block can be fatal. It can result in sudden cardiac arrest and death. This type of heart block needs emergency treatment. A temporary pacemaker may be used to keep the heart beating until you get a permanent pacemaker.

Excerpted and adapted from "Arrhythmias," July 2009, "Atrial Fibrillation," October 2009, and "Heart Block," April 2008, with supplemental information from "Long QT Syndrome," July 9, 2009, all four produced by the National Heart, Lung, and Blood Institute (NHLBI, www.nhlbi.nih.gov).

Chapter 5

Heart Murmurs and Structural Heart Disease

Sometimes birth defects or other conditions affect the function and structure of the heart.

Heart Murmur

A heart murmur is an extra or unusual sound heard during a heartbeat. Murmurs range from very faint to very loud. They sometimes sound like a whooshing or swishing noise.

Normal heartbeats make a "lub-DUPP" or "lub-DUB" sound, the sound of the heart valves closing as blood moves through the heart. Doctors can hear these sounds and heart murmurs using a stethoscope.

A heart murmur isn't a disease, and most murmurs are harmless. Innocent murmurs don't cause symptoms or require you to limit physical activity. Although an innocent murmur may be a lifelong condition, your heart is normal and you likely won't need treatment. Innocent heart murmurs are also referred to as benign heart murmurs, functional heart murmurs, physiologic heart murmurs, still murmurs, and flow murmurs.

Abnormal heart murmurs are also called pathologic heart murmurs. The outlook and treatment for abnormal heart murmurs depend on the type and severity of the heart problem causing them.

Causes of Innocent Murmurs

Innocent heart murmurs are sounds heard when blood flows through a normal heart. These murmurs may occur when blood flows faster than normal through the heart and its attached blood vessels. Illnesses or conditions that may cause this to happen include fever, anemia, and hyperthyroidism (too much thyroid hormone in the body).

Extra blood flow through the heart also may cause innocent heart murmurs. After childhood, the most common cause of extra blood flow through the heart is pregnancy. Most heart murmurs found in pregnant women are innocent. They're due to the extra blood women's bodies make while they're pregnant.

Changes to the heart that result from heart surgery or aging also may cause some innocent heart murmurs.

Causes of Abnormal Murmurs

The most common cause of abnormal murmurs in children is congenital heart defects. These are problems with the heart's structure at birth.

These defects can involve the interior walls of the heart, the valves inside the heart, or the arteries and veins that carry blood to the heart or out to the body. Some babies are born with more than one heart defect. Congenital heart defects change the normal flow of blood through the heart.

Heart valve defects and septal defects (also called holes in the heart) are common heart defects that cause abnormal heart murmurs. Valve defects may include narrow valves that limit blood flow or leaky valves that don't close properly. Septal defects are holes in the wall that separates the right and left sides of the heart. This wall is called the septum. A hole in the septum between the heart's two upper chambers is called an atrial septal defect (ASD). A hole in the septum between the heart's two lower chambers is called a ventricular septal defect (VSD). ASDs and VSDs account for more than half of all abnormal heart murmurs in children. Heart valve defects and septal defects are discussed in more detail later in this chapter.

Conditions that damage heart valves or other structures of the heart also may cause abnormal heart murmurs. These include rheumatic fever, endocarditis, calcification, and mitral valve prolapse. Heart murmurs due to these problems are more common in adults.

Signs and Symptoms

Most people who have heart murmurs don't have any other signs or symptoms of heart problems. These murmurs usually are innocent (harmless).

Some people who have heart murmurs do have signs or symptoms of heart problems. The signs and symptoms may include the following:

- Blue coloring of the skin, especially on the fingertips and inside the mouth
- Poor eating and abnormal growth (in infants)
- Shortness of breath
- Excessive sweating
- Chest pain
- Dizziness or fainting
- Fatigue

Signs and symptoms depend on the problem causing the murmur and its severity. The sections that follow discuss some of the underlying problems that may be associated with abnormal murmurs.

Holes in the Heart

Holes in the heart are simple congenital heart defects. Congenital heart defects are problems with the heart's structure at birth. These defects change the normal flow of blood through the heart.

Your heart has two sides separated by an inner wall called the septum. With each heartbeat, the right side of your heart receives oxygen-poor blood from your body and pumps it to your lungs. The left side of your heart receives oxygen-rich blood from your lungs and pumps it to your body. The septum prevents the mixing of blood between the two sides of the heart. However, some babies are born with holes in the upper or lower septum.

Over the past few decades, the diagnosis and treatment of ASDs and VSDs have greatly improved. Children who have simple congenital heart defects can survive to adulthood and live normal, active, and productive lives because their heart defects close on their own or can be repaired.

Atrial Septal Defect

An atrial septal defect is a hole in the part of the septum that separates the atria (the upper chambers of the heart). This hole allows oxygen-rich blood from the left atrium to flow into the right atrium instead of flowing into the left ventricle as it should. This means oxygen-rich blood gets pumped back to the lungs, where it has just been, instead of going to the body.

An ASD can be small or large. Small ASDs allow only a little blood to flow from one atrium to the other. Small ASDs don't affect the way the heart works and don't need any special treatment. Many small ASDs close on their own as the heart grows during childhood.

Medium to large ASDs allow more blood to leak from one atrium to the other, and they're less likely to close on their own. Most children who have ASDs have no symptoms, even if they have large ASDs.

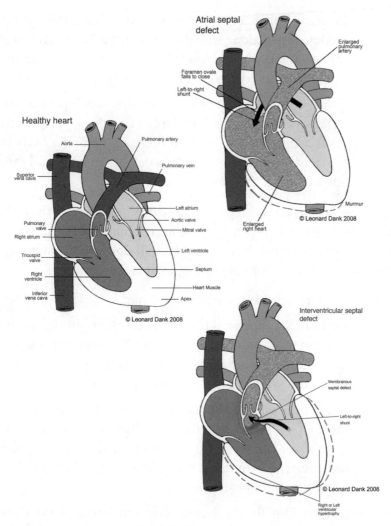

Figure 5.1. Atrial septal defect and ventricular septal defect.

There are three major types of ASDs:

- **Secundum:** This defect is in the middle of the atrial septum. It's the most common form of ASD. About 8 out of every 10 babies born with ASDs have secundum defects. At least half of all secundum ASDs close on their own. However, this is less likely if the defect is large.

- **Primum:** This defect is in the lower part of the atrial septum. It often occurs along with problems in the heart valves that connect the upper and lower heart chambers. Primum defects aren't very common, and they don't close on their own.

- **Sinus venosus:** This defect is in the upper part of the atrial septum, near where a large vein (the superior vena cava) brings oxygen-poor blood from the upper body to the right atrium. Sinus venosus defects are rare, and they don't close on their own.

Over time, if an ASD isn't repaired, the extra blood flow to the right side of the heart and lungs may cause heart problems. Usually most of these problems don't show up until adulthood, often around age 30 or later. Complications are rare in infants and children.

Possible complications include the following:

- **Right heart failure:** An ASD causes the right side of the heart to work harder because it has to pump extra blood to the lungs. Over time, the heart may become tired from this extra work and not pump well.

- **Arrhythmias:** Extra blood flowing into the right atrium through an ASD can cause the atrium to stretch and enlarge. Over time, this can lead to arrhythmias (irregular heartbeats). Arrhythmia symptoms may include palpitations or a rapid heartbeat.

- **Stroke:** Usually the lungs filter out small blood clots that can form on the right side of the heart. Sometimes a blood clot can pass from the right atrium to the left atrium through an ASD and be pumped out to the body. This type of clot can travel to an artery in the brain, block blood flow, and cause a stroke.

- **Pulmonary hypertension (PH):** PH is increased pressure in the pulmonary arteries. These arteries carry blood from your heart to your lungs to pick up oxygen. Over time, PH can damage the arteries and small blood vessels in the lungs. They become thick and stiff, making it harder for blood to flow through them.

These problems develop over many years and don't occur in children. They also are rare in adults because most ASDs either close on their own or are repaired in early childhood.

Ventricular Septal Defect

A ventricular septal defect is a hole in the part of the septum that separates the ventricles (the lower chambers of the heart). The hole allows oxygen-rich blood to flow from the left ventricle into the right ventricle instead of flowing into the aorta and out to the body as it should.

An infant who is born with a VSD may have a single hole or more than one hole in the wall that separates the two ventricles. The defect also may occur by itself or with other congenital heart defects. Doctors classify VSDs based on the size of the defect, the location of the defect, the number of defects, and the presence or absence of a ventricular septal aneurysm (a thin flap of tissue on the septum). This tissue is harmless and can help a VSD close on its own.

VSDs can be small or large. Small VSDs don't cause problems and often may close on their own. Because small VSDs allow only a small amount of blood to flow between the ventricles, they're sometimes called restrictive VSDs. Small VSDs don't cause any symptoms.

Medium VSDs are less likely to close on their own. They may require surgery to close and may cause symptoms during infancy and childhood.

Large VSDs allow a large amount of blood to flow from the left ventricle to the right ventricle. They're sometimes called nonrestrictive VSDs. A large VSD is less likely to close completely on its own, but it may get smaller over time. Large VSDs often cause symptoms in infants and children, and surgery usually is needed to close them.

VSDs are found in different parts of the septum. Membranous VSDs are located near the heart valves. These VSDs can close at any time. Muscular VSDs are found in the lower part of the septum. They're surrounded by muscle, and most close on their own during early childhood. Inlet VSDs are located close to where blood enters the ventricles. They're less common than membranous and muscular VSDs. Outlet VSDs are found in the part of the ventricle where blood leaves the heart. These are the most rare type of VSD.

Over time, if a VSD isn't repaired, it may cause heart problems. A moderate to large VSD can cause the following complications:

- **Heart failure:** Infants who have large VSDs may develop heart failure because the left side of the heart pumps blood into the right ventricle in addition to its normal work of pumping blood to the body. The increased workload on the heart also increases the heart rate and the body's demand for energy.

- **Growth failure, especially in infancy:** A baby may not be able to eat enough to keep up with his or her body's increased energy demands. As a result, the baby may lose weight or not grow and develop normally.

- **Arrhythmias (irregular heartbeats):** The extra blood flowing through the heart can cause areas of the heart to stretch and enlarge. This can disturb the heart's normal electrical activity, leading to arrhythmias.

- **PH:** The high pressure and high volume of extra blood pumped through a large VSD into the right ventricle and lungs can scar the lung's delicate arteries. Today, PH rarely develops because most large VSDs are repaired in infancy.

Causes of Septal Defects

Mothers of children who are born with atrial septal defects, ventricular septal defects, or other types of heart defects often think they did something wrong during pregnancy to cause the problems. However, most of the time, doctors don't know why congenital heart defects develop.

Heredity may play a role in some heart defects. For example, a parent who has a congenital heart defect is slightly more likely than other people to have a child with the problem. Very rarely, more than one child in a family is born with a heart defect.

Children who have genetic disorders, such as Down syndrome, often have congenital heart defects. Half of all babies who have Down syndrome have congenital heart defects.

Smoking during pregnancy also has been linked to several congenital heart defects, including septal defects.

Scientists continue to search for the causes of congenital heart defects.

ASD and VSD Signs and Symptoms

Many babies who are born with atrial septal defects have no signs or symptoms. When signs and symptoms do occur, heart murmur is the most common. Often, a heart murmur is the only sign of an ASD. However, not all murmurs are signs of congenital heart defects. Doctors can listen to heart murmurs and tell whether they're harmless or signs of heart problems.

Over time, if a large ASD isn't repaired, the extra blood flow to the right side of the heart can damage the heart and lungs and cause heart failure. This doesn't occur until adulthood. Signs and symptoms of heart failure include fatigue, tiring easily during physical activity, shortness of breath, a buildup of blood and fluid in the lungs, and a buildup of fluid in the feet, ankles, and legs.

A heart murmur usually is present in ventricular septal defect, and it may be the first and only sign of this defect. Heart murmurs often are present right after birth in many infants. However, the murmurs may not be heard until the babies are six to eight weeks old.

Most newborns who have VSDs don't have heart-related symptoms. However, babies who have medium or large VSDs can develop heart failure. Signs and symptoms of heart failure usually occur during the baby's first two months of life.

The signs and symptoms of heart failure from VSD are similar to those listed for ASD, but they occur in infancy.

A major sign of heart failure in infancy is difficulty feeding and poor growth. VSD signs and symptoms are rare after infancy because the defect either decreases in size on its own or is repaired.

Heart Valve Disease

Heart valve disease is a disease in which one or more of your heart valves don't work properly. The heart has four valves: the tricuspid, pulmonary, mitral, and aortic valves. These valves have tissue flaps that open and close with each heartbeat. The flaps make sure blood flows in the right direction through your heart's four chambers and to the rest of your body. A more detailed explanation of heart valve functioning is included in chapter 1.

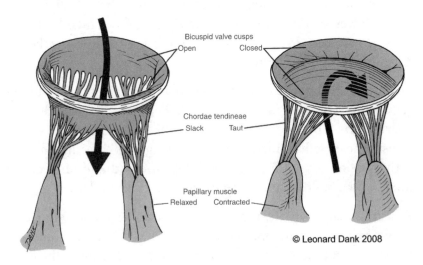

Figure 5.2. Heart valve action (mitral).

Birth defects, age-related changes, infections, or other conditions can cause one or more of your heart valves to not open fully or let blood leak back into the heart chambers. This can make your heart work harder and affect its ability to pump blood.

Types of Heart Valve Problems

Heart valves can have three basic kinds of problems: regurgitation, stenosis, and atresia.

Regurgitation, or backflow, occurs when a valve doesn't close tightly. Blood leaks back into the chambers rather than flowing forward through the heart or into an artery.

Backflow is most often due to prolapse. Prolapse is when the flaps of the valve flop or bulge back into an upper heart chamber during a heartbeat. Prolapse mainly affects the mitral valve. Mitral valve prolapse is discussed in greater detail later in this chapter.

Stenosis occurs when the flaps of a valve thicken, stiffen, or fuse together. This prevents the heart valve from fully opening. As a result, not enough blood flows through the valve. Some valves can have both stenosis and backflow problems.

Atresia occurs when a heart valve lacks an opening for blood to pass through.

You can be born with heart valve disease, or you can acquire it later in life. Heart valve disease that develops before birth is called congenital heart valve disease. Congenital heart valve disease can occur alone or with other congenital heart defects.

Congenital heart valve disease usually involves pulmonary or aortic valves that don't form properly. These valves may not have enough tissue flaps, they may be the wrong size or shape, or they may lack an opening through which blood can flow properly.

Acquired heart valve disease usually involves the aortic or mitral valve. Although the valve is normal at first, the disease can cause problems to develop over time.

Both congenital and acquired heart valve disease can cause stenosis or backflow.

Many people have heart valve defects or disease but don't have symptoms. For some people, the condition mostly stays the same throughout their lives and doesn't cause any problems.

For other people, the condition slowly worsens until symptoms develop. If not treated, advanced heart valve disease can cause heart failure, stroke, blood clots, or sudden death due to sudden cardiac arrest.

Currently, no medicines can cure heart valve disease. However, lifestyle changes and medicines can relieve many of the symptoms and problems linked to heart valve disease. These treatments also can lower your risk of developing a life-threatening condition, such as stroke or sudden cardiac arrest. Eventually, a faulty heart valve may need to be repaired or replaced.

Some types of congenital heart valve disease are so severe that the valve is repaired or replaced during infancy, childhood, or even before birth. Other types may not cause problems until you're middle-aged or older, if at all.

Other Names for Types of Heart Valve Disease

- Aortic regurgitation
- Aortic stenosis
- Aortic sclerosis
- Bicuspid aortic valve
- Mitral regurgitation
- Mitral stenosis
- Mitral valve prolapse
- Pulmonic regurgitation
- Pulmonic stenosis
- Tricuspid regurgitation
- Tricuspid stenosis

Causes

The cause of congenital heart valve disease isn't known. It occurs before birth as the heart is forming. Congenital heart valve disease can occur alone or with other types of congenital heart defects.

Heart conditions and other disorders, age-related changes, rheumatic fever, and infections can cause acquired heart valve disease. These factors change the shape or flexibility of once-normal valves.

Heart valves can be stretched and distorted by damage or scar tissue from a heart attack or injury to the heart. Advanced high blood pressure and heart failure can also damage heart valves (these conditions can enlarge the heart or the main arteries). Also, narrowing of the aorta due to the buildup of a fatty material called plaque inside the artery can lead to heart valve disease. (The aorta is the main artery that carries oxygen-rich blood to the body. When plaque builds up inside the arteries, the condition is called atherosclerosis.)

Men older than 65 and women older than 75 are prone to developing calcium deposits and other deposits on their heart valves. These deposits stiffen and thicken the valve flaps and limit blood flow (stenosis). The aortic valve is especially prone to this problem. The deposits resemble those seen in the narrowed and hardened blood vessels of people who have atherosclerosis. Some of the same processes may cause both atherosclerosis and heart valve disease.

Some people have heart valve disease due to rheumatic fever, a rare complication of certain strep infections. Other infections can also play a role in heart valve disease. Common germs that enter the bloodstream and get carried to the heart can sometimes infect the inner surface of the heart, including the heart valves. This rare, but sometimes life-threatening, infection is called infective endocarditis, or IE. (For more on heart infections, see chapter 6.)

A number of other conditions and factors are sometimes linked to heart valve disease. However, it's often unknown how these conditions actually cause heart valve disease.

- **Lupus:** Lupus and other immune diseases can affect the aortic and mitral valves.

- **Carcinoid syndrome:** Tumors in the digestive tract that spread to the liver or lymph nodes can affect the tricuspid and pulmonary valves.

- **Metabolic disorders:** Relatively uncommon diseases, such as Fabry disease and hyperlipidemia, can affect the heart valves.

- **Diet medicines:** The use of fenfluramine and phentermine (fen-phen) has sometimes been linked to heart valve problems. These problems typically stabilize or improve after the medicine is stopped.

- **Radiation therapy:** Radiation therapy to the chest area can cause heart valve disease. This therapy is used to treat cancer. Heart valve disease due to radiation therapy may not cause symptoms for as many as 20 years after the therapy ends.

- **Marfan syndrome:** Congenital disorders, such as Marfan syndrome and other connective tissue disorders, mainly affect the structure of the body's main arteries. However, these conditions also can affect the heart valves.

Signs and Symptoms

The main sign of heart valve disease is a heart murmur; however, as noted previously, many people have heart murmurs without having heart valve disease or any other heart problems. Others may have heart murmurs due to heart valve disease but no other signs or symptoms.

Heart valve disease often worsens over time, so signs and symptoms may develop years after a heart murmur is first heard. Many people who have heart valve disease don't have any symptoms until they're middle-aged or older.

Other common signs and symptoms of heart valve disease relate to heart failure, which heart valve disease can eventually cause. These symptoms include unusual fatigue, shortness of breath (especially when you exert yourself or when you're lying down), and swelling in your ankles, feet, legs, abdomen, and the veins in your neck.

Heart valve disease can cause chest pain that may only occur when you exert yourself. You also may notice a fluttering, racing, or irregular heartbeat. Some types of heart valve disease, such as aortic or mitral valve stenosis, can cause dizziness or fainting.

Mitral Valve Prolapse

Mitral valve prolapse (MVP) is a condition in which one of the heart's valves, the mitral valve, doesn't work properly. The flaps of the valve are floppy and don't close tightly. MVP is also sometimes referred to as Barlow syndrome, click-murmur syndrome, or floppy valve syndrome.

Much of the time, MVP doesn't cause any problems. Rarely, blood can leak the wrong way through the floppy valve, which may cause shortness of breath, palpitations (strong or rapid heartbeats), chest pain, and other symptoms.

Normal Mitral Valve

The mitral valve controls the flow of blood between the two chambers on the left side of the heart. The two chambers are the left atrium and the left ventricle.

The mitral valve allows blood to flow from the left atrium to the left ventricle but not back the other way. (The heart also has a right atrium and ventricle, separated by the tricuspid valve.)

At the beginning of a heartbeat, the atria contract and push blood through to the ventricles. The flaps of the mitral and tricuspid valves swing open to let the blood through. Then the ventricles contract to pump the blood out of the heart.

When the ventricles contract, the flaps of the mitral and tricuspid valves swing shut. They form a tight seal that prevents blood from flowing back into the atria.

What Goes Wrong

In MVP, when the left ventricle contracts, one or both flaps of the mitral valve flop or bulge back (prolapse) into the left atrium. This can prevent the valve from forming a tight seal.

As a result, blood may flow backward from the ventricle into the atrium. The backflow of blood is called regurgitation.

Backflow doesn't occur in all cases of MVP. In fact, most people who have MVP don't have backflow and never have any symptoms or complications. In these people, even though the valve flaps prolapse, the valve still can form a tight seal.

When backflow does occur, it can cause symptoms and complications such as shortness of breath, arrhythmias, or chest pain. For more information about arrhythmias—problems with the rate or rhythm of the heartbeat—see chapter 4.

Backflow can get worse over time. It can lead to changes in the heart's size and higher pressures in the left atrium and lungs. Backflow also increases the risk for heart valve infections. Rarely, MVP can cause infective endocarditis, discussed in chapter 6.

A small number of people who have MVP may need medicines to relieve their symptoms. Very few people who have MVP need heart valve surgery to repair their mitral valves.

MVP was once thought to affect as much as 5 to 15% of the population. It's now believed that many people who were diagnosed with

MVP in the past didn't actually have an abnormal mitral valve. They may have had a slight bulging of the valve flaps due to other conditions, such as dehydration or a small heart. However, their valves were normal, and there was little or no backflow of blood through their valves.

Now, diagnosing MVP is more precise because of a test called echocardiography, which allows doctors to easily identify true MVP and detect troublesome backflow. As a result, it's now believed that less than 3% of the population actually has true MVP, and an even smaller percentage has serious complications from it.

Most people who have MVP have no symptoms or medical problems and don't need treatment. These people are able to lead normal, active lives; they may not even know they have the condition.

Causes

The exact cause of mitral valve prolapse isn't known. Most people who have the condition are born with it. MVP tends to run in families and is more common in people born with connective tissue disorders, such as Marfan syndrome.

The mitral valve can be abnormal in two ways. First, the valve flaps may be oversized and thickened. Second, the valve flaps may be floppy. The tissue of the flaps and their supporting "strings" are too stretchy, and parts of the valve flop or bulge back into the atrium.

Some people's valves are abnormal in both ways. Either way can keep the valve from making a tight seal.

Signs and Symptoms

Most people who have mitral valve prolapse aren't affected by the condition because they don't have any symptoms or major mitral valve backflow. Among those who do have symptoms, palpitations (strong or rapid heartbeats) are reported most often. Other symptoms include shortness of breath, cough, dizziness, fatigue, anxiety, migraine headaches, and chest discomfort.

MVP symptoms can vary from one person to another. They tend to be mild but can worsen over time, mainly when complications occur.

Complications

Complications of MVP are rare. When present, they're most often due to the backflow of blood through the mitral valve. Mitral valve backflow causes blood to flow backward from the left ventricle into the left atrium. Blood can even back up from the atrium into the lungs, causing shortness of breath.

Mitral valve backflow is most common among men and people who have high blood pressure. People who have severe cases of backflow may need valve surgery to prevent complications.

The backflow of blood puts a strain on the muscles of both the atrium and the ventricle. Over time, the strain can lead to arrhythmias. One troublesome arrhythmia caused by MVP is atrial fibrillation. This condition, and other arrhythmias, are discussed in chapter 4.

Infection of the mitral valve is another complication of MVP. A deformed mitral valve flap attracts bacteria that may be in the bloodstream. The bacteria attach to the valve and can cause a serious infection called infective endocarditis.

Excerpted and adapted from "Heart Murmur," June 2008, "Heart Valve Disease," January 2010, "Holes in the Heart," October 2009, and "Mitral Valve Prolapse," July 2009, all four produced by the National Heart, Lung, and Blood Institute (NHLBI, www.nhlbi.nih.gov).

Chapter 6

Heart Infections

Endocarditis

Endocarditis is an infection of the inner lining of your heart chambers and valves. This lining is called the endocardium. The condition is called infective endocarditis (IE).

The term *endocarditis* also is used to describe an inflammation of the endocardium due to other conditions. This chapter discusses endocarditis related to infection.

IE can develop quickly or slowly depending on what type of germ is causing it and whether you have an underlying heart problem. When IE develops quickly, it's called acute infective endocarditis. When it develops slowly, it's called subacute infective endocarditis.

Infective endocarditis causes a range of signs and symptoms that can vary from person to person. Signs and symptoms also can vary over time in the same person. If you have signs or symptoms of IE, you should see your doctor as soon as you can, especially if you have abnormal heart valves.

Signs and symptoms differ depending on whether you have an underlying heart problem, the type of germ causing the infection, and whether you have acute or subacute IE. The signs and symptoms of IE may include the following:

- Flu-like symptoms, such as fever, chills, fatigue, aching muscles and joints, night sweats, and headache
- Shortness of breath or a cough that won't go away
- A new heart murmur or a change in an existing heart murmur
- Skin changes such as overall paleness; small, painful, red or purplish bumps under the skin on the fingers or toes; small, dark, painless, flat spots on the palms of the hands or the soles of the feet; and tiny spots under the fingernails, on the whites of the eyes, on the roof of the mouth and inside of the cheeks, or on the chest (these spots are from broken blood vessels)
- Nausea, vomiting, a decrease in appetite, a sense of fullness with discomfort on the upper left side of the abdomen, or weight loss with or without a change in appetite
- Blood in the urine
- Swelling in the feet, legs, or abdomen

IE Causes

Infective endocarditis is an uncommon condition that can affect both children and adults. It's more common in men than women.

IE occurs when bacteria, fungi, or other germs invade your bloodstream and attach to abnormal areas of your heart. Certain factors increase the risk of germs attaching to a heart valve or chamber and causing an infection.

IE typically affects people who have abnormal hearts or other conditions that make them more likely to get the infection, but in some cases IE affects people who were healthy before the infection. A common underlying factor in IE is a structural heart defect, especially faulty heart valves. Usually your immune system will kill germs in your bloodstream. However, if your heart has a rough lining or abnormal valves, the invading germs can attach and multiply in the heart. The germs that cause IE tend to attach and multiply on damaged, malformed, or artificial heart valves and implanted medical devices.

Other factors, such as those that allow germs to build up in your bloodstream, also can play a role in causing IE. Common activities, such as brushing your teeth or having certain dental procedures, can allow bacteria to enter your bloodstream. This is more likely to happen if your teeth and gums are in poor condition.

Having a catheter or another medical device inserted through your skin, especially for long periods, also can allow bacteria to enter your bloodstream. People who use intravenous drugs also are at risk for infections due to germs on needles and syringes.

Bacteria also may spread to the blood and heart from infections in other parts of the body, such as the gut, skin, or genitals.

Complications

As bacteria or other germs multiply in your heart, they form clumps with other cells and matter found in the blood. These clumps are called vegetations.

As IE worsens, pieces of these vegetations can break off and travel to almost any other organ or tissue in the body. There the pieces can block blood flow or cause a new infection. As a result, IE can cause a wide range of complications.

Heart problems are the most common complication of IE. They occur in one-third to one-half of all people who have the infection. These problems may include a new heart murmur, heart failure, heart valve damage, heart block, or, rarely, a heart attack.

Infective Endocarditis and Dental Work

A link has long been suspected between dental procedures and infective endocarditis. Many cases of infective endocarditis are caused by types of bacteria that live in the mouth and on teeth. Experiments have shown that dental cleaning and some other procedures can cause oral bacteria to be briefly detectable in the blood. Additionally, a number of patients have reported undergoing dental procedures in the weeks prior to developing infective endocarditis.

For many years, most people with heart murmurs were advised to take doses of antibiotics before dental cleaning and other procedures. The hope was this would kill bacteria that entered the blood during dental work.

While this practice was widely recommended by authorities in the field, some scientists criticized the strategy. They pointed to the fact that no study has ever actually proven a relationship between dental cleaning and actual cases of infective endocarditis. Experiments showed bacteria also entered the blood after normal eating and routine toothbrushing. Finally, there were no studies showing that giving antibiotics before dental work actually reduced the risk of developing infective endocarditis.

However, in 2008, the American Heart Association, the American College of Cardiology, and the American Dental Association reversed their position on giving antibiotics before dental work. They conceded that available scientific evidence did not support routine treatment with antibiotics before dental cleaning. Additionally, there was concern that even if the strategy was effective, treating millions of people with antibiotics probably caused more complications from antibiotic use than the number of cases of endocarditis it prevented.

Currently, taking antibiotics before dental work for the prevention of infectious endocarditis is only recommended for the patients at highest risk: those with mechanical heart valves, certain corrective procedures for congenital heart disease, or who have previously had infectious endocarditis. The vast majority of people with heart murmurs or valve disease are no longer recommended to take antibiotics before dental work.

If you had been previously advised to take antibiotics before dental work, you should ask your doctor whether you still should be doing so.

Central nervous system complications occur in as many as 20 to 40% of people who have IE. Central nervous system complications most often occur when bits of vegetation, called emboli, break away and lodge in the brain. There they can cause local infections (called brain abscesses) or a more widespread brain infection (called meningitis).

Emboli also can cause a stroke or seizures. This happens if they block blood vessels or affect the brain's electrical signals. These complications can cause long-lasting damage to the brain and may even be fatal.

IE also can affect other organs in the body, such as the lungs, kidneys, and spleen:

- **Lungs:** The lungs are especially at risk when IE affects the right side of the heart. This is called right-sided infective endocarditis. A vegetation or blood clot going to the lungs can cause a pulmonary embolism and lung damage. Other lung complications include pneumonia and a buildup of fluid or pus around the lungs.

- **Kidneys:** IE can cause kidney abscesses and kidney damage. IE also can cause inflammation of the internal filtering structures of the kidneys. Signs and symptoms of kidney complications include back or side pain, blood in the urine, and a change in the color or amount of urine. In a small number of people, IE can cause kidney failure.

- **Spleen:** The spleen is an organ located in the left upper part of the abdomen near the stomach. In as many as 25 to 60% of people who have IE, the spleen enlarges (especially in people who have long-term IE). Sometimes, emboli also can damage the spleen. Signs and symptoms of spleen problems include pain or discomfort in the upper left abdomen and/or left shoulder, a feeling of fullness or the inability to eat large meals, and hiccups.

Pericarditis

Pericarditis is a condition in which the membrane, or sac, around your heart is inflamed. This sac is called the pericardium.

The pericardium holds the heart in place and helps it work properly. The sac is made of two thin layers of tissue that enclose your heart. Between the two layers is a small amount of fluid. This fluid keeps the layers from rubbing against each other and causing friction.

In pericarditis, the layers of tissue become inflamed and can rub against the heart. This causes chest pain—a common symptom of pericarditis.

It may take from a few days to weeks or even months to recover from pericarditis. With proper and prompt treatment, such as rest and ongoing care, most people make a full recovery. These measures also can help reduce the chances of getting the condition again.

Causes

There are several types of pericarditis. Acute pericarditis occurs suddenly; chronic pericarditis develops and persists over time. The causes of acute and chronic pericarditis are the same, but the cause of about half of all pericarditis cases (both acute and chronic) is unknown. The term *idiopathic pericarditis* refers to pericarditis with no known cause.

Viral infections are likely the most common cause of acute pericarditis, but the virus may never be found. Pericarditis often occurs after a respiratory infection. Bacterial, fungal, and other infections also can cause pericarditis. Less often, pericarditis may be caused by other conditions:

- Autoimmune disorders, such as lupus, scleroderma, and rheumatoid arthritis

- Heart attack and heart surgery

- Kidney failure, HIV/AIDS, cancer, tuberculosis, and other health problems

- Injury from accidents or radiation therapy

- Certain medicines, like phenytoin (an antiseizure medicine), warfarin and heparin (blood-thinning medicines), and pro-cainamide (a medicine to treat abnormal heartbeats)

- Some cancers may spread to the pericardium, and coat the inside of the sac. This may be referred to as carci-nomatous pericarditis. This can lead to substantial fluid buildup inside the pericardium.

Signs and Symptoms

Sharp, stabbing chest pain is a common symptom of acute pericardi-tis. The pain usually comes on quickly. It often is felt in the middle or the left side of the chest. The pain tends to ease when you sit up and lean forward. Lying down and breathing deep worsens it. For some people, the pain feels like a dull ache or pressure in their chest.

The chest pain may feel like pain from a heart attack. If you have chest pain, you should call 911 right away, as you may be having a heart attack.

Fever is another common symptom of acute pericarditis. Other symptoms are weakness, trouble breathing, and coughing.

Chronic pericarditis often causes tiredness, coughing, and short-ness of breath. Chest pain is often absent in this type of pericardi-tis. Severe cases of chronic pericarditis can lead to swelling in the stomach and legs and low blood pressure (hypotension).

Complications

Two serious complications of pericarditis are cardiac tamponade and chronic constrictive pericarditis.

Cardiac tamponade occurs when too much fluid collects in the pericardium. The extra fluid puts pressure on the heart. This pre-vents the heart from properly filling with blood. As a result, less blood leaves the heart. This causes a sharp drop in blood pressure. If left untreated, cardiac tamponade can cause death.

Chronic constrictive pericarditis is a rare disease that develops over time. It leads to scar-like tissue throughout the pericardium. The sac becomes stiff and can't move properly. In time, the scarred tissue compresses the heart and prevents it from working correctly.

Excerpted and adapted from "Endocarditis," November 2008, and "Pericarditis," March 2008, both produced by the National Heart, Lung, and Blood Institute (NHLBI, www.nhlbi.nih.gov), with supplemental information about antibiotics and endocarditis added by David A. Cooke, MD, FACP, May 2010.

Chapter 7

Aortic Aneurysm

The major artery leaving the heart is called the aorta. When your heart pumps, it sends oxygen-rich blood through the aorta to the rest of your body by way of a branching system of arteries.

Arteries have thick walls to withstand normal blood pressure. However, certain medical problems, genetic conditions, and trauma can damage or injure artery walls. An aneurysm is a balloon-like bulge in an artery. The force of blood pushing against the weakened or injured walls can cause an aneurysm.

An aneurysm can grow large and burst, which is called a rupture. Rupture causes dangerous bleeding inside the body. An aneurysm can also cause a dissection—a split in one or more layers of the artery wall. The split causes bleeding into and along the layers of the artery wall. Both conditions are often fatal.

There are two types of aneurysm that affect the aorta: abdominal aortic aneurysm (AAA) and thoracic aortic aneurysm (TAA). When found in time, aortic aneurysms often can be successfully treated with medicines or surgery.

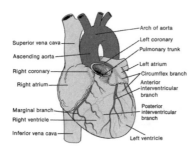

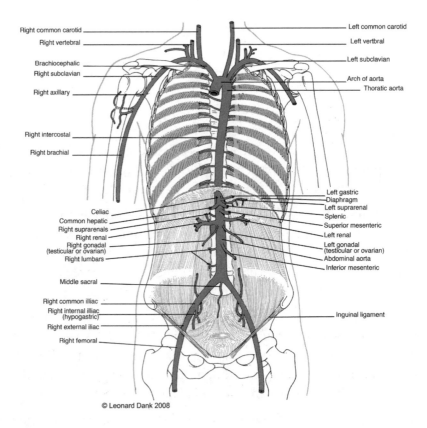

© Leonard Dank 2008

Figure 7.1. Coronary arteries and major arteries of the chest.

Abdominal Aortic Aneurysms

An aneurysm that occurs in the part of the aorta that's located in the abdomen is called an abdominal aortic aneurysm. AAAs account for three in four aortic aneurysms. They're found more often now than in the past because of computed tomography (CT) scans done for other medical problems.

Small AAAs rarely rupture. However, an AAA can grow very large without causing symptoms. Thus, routine checkups and treatment for an AAA are important to prevent growth and rupture.

Thoracic Aortic Aneurysms

An aneurysm that occurs in the part of the aorta that's located in the chest and above the diaphragm is called a thoracic aortic aneurysm. TAAs account for one in four aortic aneurysms.

TAAs don't always cause symptoms, even when they're large. Only half of all people who have TAAs notice any symptoms.

With a common type of TAA, the walls of the aorta weaken, and a section close to the heart enlarges. As a result, the valve between the heart and the aorta can't close properly, which allows blood to leak back into the heart.

A less common type of TAA can develop in the upper back, away from the heart. A TAA in this location may result from an injury to the chest, such as from a car crash.

Other Types of Aneurysms

Aneurysms can also occur in other arteries. When an aneurysm occurs in an artery in the brain, it's called a cerebral aneurysm or brain aneurysm. Brain aneurysms also are sometimes called berry aneurysms because they're often the size of a small berry. Most brain aneurysms cause no symptoms until they become large, begin to leak blood, or rupture. A ruptured brain aneurysm causes a stroke.

Aneurysms that occur in arteries other than the aorta and the brain arteries are called peripheral aneurysms. Common locations for peripheral aneurysms include the popliteal, femoral, and carotid arteries. The popliteal arteries run down the back of the thighs, behind the knees. The femoral arteries are the main arteries in the groin. The carotid arteries are the main arteries on each side of your neck.

Peripheral aneurysms aren't as likely to rupture or dissect as aortic aneurysms. However, blood clots can form in peripheral aneurysms. If a blood clot breaks away from the aneurysm, it can block blood flow through the artery. If a peripheral aneurysm is large, it can press on a nearby nerve or vein and cause pain, numbness, or swelling.

Causes of Aortic Aneurysms

A number of factors can damage and weaken the walls of the aorta and cause aortic aneurysms. Aging, smoking, high blood pressure, and atherosclerosis are all risk factors. Rarely, infections, such as untreated syphilis (a sexually transmitted infection), can cause aortic aneurysms. Aortic aneurysms also can occur as a result of diseases that inflame the blood vessels, such as vasculitis. Family history also may play a role in causing aortic aneurysms.

In addition, certain genetic conditions may cause thoracic aortic aneurysms. Examples include Marfan syndrome, Loeys-Dietz syndrome, and Ehlers-Danlos syndrome (the vascular type). These conditions can weaken the body's connective tissues and damage the aorta. People who have these conditions tend to develop aneurysms at a younger age and are at higher risk for rupture or dissection.

Trauma, such as a car accident, also can damage the aorta walls and lead to TAAs.

Researchers continue to look for other causes of aortic aneurysms. For example, they're looking for genetic mutations that may contribute to or cause aneurysms.

Signs and Symptoms

The signs and symptoms of an aortic aneurysm depend on the type of aneurysm, its location, and whether it has ruptured or is affecting other parts of the body.

Aneurysms can develop and grow for years without causing any signs or symptoms. They often don't cause signs or symptoms until they rupture, grow large enough to press on nearby parts of the body, or block blood flow.

Most abdominal aortic aneurysms develop slowly over years. Most often, they don't have signs or symptoms unless they rupture. If you have an AAA, your doctor may feel a throbbing mass while checking your abdomen. Possible symptoms include a throbbing feeling in the abdomen, deep pain in your back or the side of your abdomen, and a steady, gnawing pain in your abdomen that lasts for hours or days.

If an AAA ruptures, symptoms can include sudden, severe pain in your lower abdomen and back; nausea and vomiting; clammy, sweaty skin; light-headedness; and a rapid heart rate when standing up. Internal bleeding from a ruptured AAA can send you into shock. Shock is a life-threatening condition in which the body's organs don't get enough blood flow. It requires emergency treatment.

A thoracic aortic aneurysm may not cause symptoms until it dissects or grows large. At this point, symptoms may include pain in your jaw, neck, back, or chest and coughing, hoarseness, or trouble breathing or swallowing.

If a TAA ruptures or dissects, you may feel sudden, severe pain starting in your upper back and moving down into your abdomen. You may have pain in your chest and arms, and you can quickly go into shock.

If you have any symptoms of TAA or aortic dissection, call 911. If left untreated, these conditions may lead to organ damage or death.

Excerpted and adapted from "Aneurysm," National Heart, Lung, and Blood Institute (NHLBI, www.nhlbi.nih.gov), April 2009.

Part Two

Tests, Procedures, and Treatments

Finding out you have heart disease is the beginning of your journey back to wellness. This part discusses the tools your doctor may use to clarify your diagnosis, check for other problems, and treat or monitor your condition.

First, you'll find information about various blood tests your doctor may use to assess risks to your heart's health or learn about how your muscles and organs are functioning. Then, several chapters offer detailed information about methods to determine exactly how your heart is working and what is causing any problems.

Electrocardiography and stress testing are tests that gather information about your heart by measuring its electrical activity and response to physical stress. Holter and event monitors serve a similar purpose, but they enable your doctor to record what your heart is doing as you go about your normal daily routine.

Echocardiography has a different function. It uses sound waves to create an image that lets your doctor see how well your heart's muscles, valves, and chambers are functioning. Nuclear heart scanning, computed tomography, and magnetic resonance imaging are other methods for obtaining different images of your heart.

Sometimes your doctor may need images of the inside of your arteries, which involves a test called coronary angiography. It uses special x-rays to create an image of the insides of your arteries. The test involves placing a dye into your bloodstream using a procedure called cardiac catheterization. The process of catheterization can also be used as part of a treatment procedure for opening blocked arteries or treating some types of arrhythmia.

In addition to these tests, your doctor may want you to take certain medicines. Some people with heart disease benefit from taking a daily dose of aspirin. Some take blood thinners to reduce the risk of heart attacks from blood clots. Others use medications or dietary supplements to manage blood pressure or blood cholesterol. Individual chapters address the benefits and risks of the most commonly used heart medications.

Not all heart problems can be fixed with medicines, however. Every year in the United States, more than half a million people undergo surgical procedures to address heart problems that haven't responded to other, less invasive treatments. This part of the book concludes with a group of chapters that discuss the most commonly performed heart surgeries, including angioplasty, coronary artery bypass grafting, the implantation of devices to help regulate heart rhythm, and transplants.

Chapter 8

Common Blood Tests

Understanding Blood Tests

Blood tests help doctors check for certain diseases and conditions. Specifically, blood tests can help doctors evaluate how well organs, like the kidneys, liver, and heart, are working or diagnose diseases and conditions such as cancer, HIV/AIDS, diabetes, anemia, and coronary heart disease (also called coronary artery disease). Blood tests can also help doctors learn whether you have risk factors for heart disease or check whether medicines you're taking are working. Some of the most common blood tests include a complete blood count (CBC), blood chemistry tests, blood enzyme tests, and blood tests to assess heart disease risk.

Many blood tests don't require any special preparations. For some, you may need to fast (not eat any food) for 8 to 12 hours before the test. Your doctor will let you know how to prepare for blood tests.

During a blood test, a small amount of blood is taken from your body. It's usually drawn from a vein in your arm using a needle.

A finger prick also may be used. The procedure usually is quick and easy, although it may cause some short-term discomfort. Most people don't have serious reactions to having blood drawn.

Lab workers draw the blood and analyze it. They use either whole blood to count blood cells or separate the blood cells from the fluid that contains them. This fluid is called plasma or serum.

The fluid is used to measure different substances in the blood. The results can help detect health problems in their early stages, when treatments or lifestyle changes may work best.

However, blood tests alone can't be used to diagnose many diseases or medical problems. Your doctor may consider other factors, such as your signs and symptoms, your medical history, and results from other tests and procedures, to confirm a diagnosis.

Blood tests have few risks. Most complications are minor and go away shortly after the tests are done.

Complete Blood Count

The CBC is one of the most common blood tests. It's often done as part of a routine checkup. The CBC can help detect blood diseases and disorders, such as anemia, infections, clotting problems, blood cancers, and immune system disorders. This test measures many different parts of your blood.

Red Blood Cells

Red blood cells carry oxygen from your lungs to the rest of your body. Abnormal red blood cell levels may be a sign of anemia, dehydration (too little fluid in the body), bleeding, or another disorder.

White Blood Cells

White blood cells are part of your immune system, which fights infections and diseases. Abnormal white blood cell levels may be a sign of infection, blood cancer, or an immune system disorder.

A CBC measures the overall number of white blood cells in your blood. A CBC with differential looks at the amounts of different types of white blood cells in your blood.

Platelets

Platelets are blood cell fragments that help your blood clot. They stick together to seal cuts or breaks on blood vessel walls and stop bleeding.

Abnormal platelet levels may be a sign of a bleeding disorder (not enough clotting) or a thrombotic disorder (too much clotting).

Hemoglobin

Hemoglobin is an iron-rich protein in red blood cells that carries oxygen. Abnormal hemoglobin levels may be a sign of anemia, sickle cell anemia, thalassemia, or other blood disorders.

If you have diabetes, excess glucose in your blood can attach to hemoglobin and raise the level of hemoglobin A1c.

Hematocrit

Hematocrit is a measure of how much space red blood cells take up in your blood. A high hematocrit level might mean you're dehydrated. A low hematocrit level might mean you have anemia. Abnormal hematocrit levels also may be a sign of a blood or bone marrow disorder.

Mean Corpuscular Volume

Mean corpuscular volume (MCV) is a measure of the average size of your red blood cells. Abnormal MCV levels may be a sign of anemia or thalassemia.

Blood Chemistry Tests/Basic Metabolic Panel

The basic metabolic panel (BMP) is a group of tests that measures different chemicals in the blood. These tests usually are done on the fluid (plasma) part of the blood. BMP tests can give doctors information about your muscles (including the heart), bones, and organs, such as the kidneys and liver.

The BMP includes blood glucose, calcium, and electrolyte tests, as well as blood tests that measure kidney function. Some of these tests require you to fast before the test, and others don't. Your doctor will tell you how to prepare for the test(s) you're having.

Blood Glucose

Glucose is a type of sugar the body uses for energy. Abnormal glucose levels in your blood may be a sign of diabetes.

For some blood glucose tests, you have to fast before your blood is drawn. Other blood glucose tests are done after a meal or at any time with no preparation.

Calcium

Calcium is an important mineral in the body. Abnormal calcium levels in the blood may be a sign of kidney problems, bone disease, thyroid disease, cancer, malnutrition, or another disorder.

Electrolytes

Electrolytes are minerals that help maintain fluid levels and acid-base balance in the body. They include sodium, potassium, bicarbonate, and chloride.

Abnormal electrolyte levels may be a sign of dehydration, kidney disease, liver disease, heart failure, high blood pressure, or other disorders.

Kidneys

Blood tests for kidney function measure levels of blood urea nitrogen (BUN) and creatinine. Both are waste products the kidneys filter out of the body. Abnormal BUN and creatinine levels may be signs of a kidney disease or disorder.

Blood Enzyme Tests

Enzymes are chemicals that help control chemical reactions in your body. There are many blood enzyme tests. This section focuses on blood enzyme tests used to check for heart attack. These include troponin and creatine kinase (CK) tests.

Troponin

Troponin is a muscle protein that helps your muscles contract. When muscle or heart cells are injured, troponin leaks out, and its levels in your blood rise. For example, blood levels of troponin rise when you have a heart attack. For this reason, doctors often order troponin tests when patients have chest pain or other heart attack signs and symptoms.

Creatine Kinase

A blood product called CK-MB is released when the heart muscle is damaged. High levels of CK-MB in the blood can mean that you've had a heart attack.

Blood Tests to Assess Heart Disease Risk

A lipoprotein panel is a blood test that can help show whether you're at risk for coronary heart disease (CHD). This test looks at substances in your blood that carry cholesterol. A lipoprotein panel displays information about the following things:

- **Total cholesterol**

- **Low-density lipoprotein (LDL, or bad) cholesterol:** This is the main source of cholesterol buildup and blockages in the arteries.

- **High-density lipoprotein (HDL, or good) cholesterol:** This type of cholesterol helps decrease blockages in the arteries.

- **Triglycerides:** Triglycerides are a type of fat in your blood.

Most people will need to fast for 9 to 12 hours before a lipoprotein panel. Abnormal cholesterol and triglyceride levels may be signs of increased risk for CHD.

What to Expect from Blood Tests

What to Expect during Blood Tests

Blood usually is drawn from a vein in your arm or other part of your body using a needle. It also can be drawn using a finger prick.

The person who draws your blood might tie a band around the upper part of your arm or ask you to make a fist. This can make the veins in your arm stick out more, which makes it easier to insert the needle.

The needle that goes into your vein is attached to a small test tube. The person who draws your blood removes the tube when it's full, and the tube seals on its own. The needle is then removed from your vein. If you're getting a few blood tests, more than one test tube may be attached to the needle before it's withdrawn.

Some people get nervous about blood tests because they're afraid of needles. Others may not want to see blood leaving their bodies. If you're nervous or scared, it can help to look away or talk to someone to distract yourself. You might feel a slight sting when the needle goes in or comes out.

Drawing blood usually takes less than three minutes.

What to Expect after Blood Tests

Once the needle is withdrawn, you'll be asked to apply gentle pressure with a piece of gauze or bandage to the place where the needle was inserted. This helps stop bleeding and prevents swelling and bruising.

Most of the time, you can remove the pressure after a minute or two. You may want to keep a bandage on for a few hours.

Usually you don't need to do anything else after a blood test. Results can take anywhere from a few minutes to a few weeks. Your doctor should get the results. It's important to follow up with your doctor to discuss your test results.

Blood Test Risks

The main risks of blood tests are discomfort and bruising at the site of the needle puncture. These complications usually are minor and go away shortly after the tests are done.

Blood Test Results

Blood tests show whether the levels of different substances in your blood fall within a normal range.

For many blood substances, the normal range is the range of levels seen in 95% of healthy people in a certain group. For many tests, normal ranges are different depending on your age, gender, race, and other factors.

Many factors can cause your blood test levels to fall outside the normal range. Abnormal levels may be a sign of a disorder or disease. Other factors—such as diet, menstrual cycle, physical activity, alcohol consumption, and the medicines you take (both prescription and over-the-counter)—also can cause abnormal levels.

Your doctor should discuss any unusual or abnormal blood test results with you. These results may or may not suggest a health problem.

Blood tests alone can't be used to diagnose many diseases or medical problems. However, blood tests can help you and your doctor learn more about your health. Blood tests also can help find potential problems early, when treatments or lifestyle changes may work best.

Result Ranges for Common Blood Tests

This section presents the result ranges for some of the most common blood tests. It is important to note that all values in this section are for adults only. They don't apply to children. Talk to your child's doctor about values on blood tests for children.

Complete Blood Count

Table 8.1 shows some normal ranges for different parts of the CBC. Some of the normal ranges are different for men and women. Other factors, such as age and race, also may affect normal ranges.

Your doctor should discuss your results with you. He or she will advise you further if your results are outside the normal range for your group.

Table 8.1. Result Ranges for Complete Blood Count

Test	Normal Range Results
Red blood cell (varies with altitude)	Male: 5 to 6 million cells/mcL Female: 4 to 5 million cells/mcL
White blood cell	4,500 to 10,000 cells/mcL
Platelets	140,000 to 450,000 cells/mcL
Hemoglobin (varies with altitude)	Male: 14 to 17 gm/dL Female: 12 to 15 gm/dL
Hematocrit (varies with altitude)	Male: 41% to 50% Female: 36% to 44%
Mean corpuscular volume	80 to 95 femtoliter

Note: cells/mcL = cells per microliter; gm/dL = grams per deciliter.

Table 8.2. Result Ranges for Plasma Glucose Test

Plasma Glucose Results (mg/dL)[a]	Diagnosis
99 and below	Normal
100 to 125	Prediabetes
126 and above	Diabetes[b]

[a]mg/dL = milligrams per deciliter.

[b]If the result indicates diabetes, the test is repeated on another day to confirm the results.

Blood Glucose

Table 8.2 shows the ranges for blood glucose levels after 8 to 12 hours of fasting (not eating). It shows the normal range and the abnormal ranges that are a sign of prediabetes or diabetes.

Lipoprotein Panel

Table 8.3 shows ranges for total cholesterol, LDL cholesterol, and HDL cholesterol levels after 9 to 12 hours of fasting. High blood cholesterol is a risk factor for coronary heart disease.

Your doctor should discuss your results with you. He or she will advise you further if your results are outside the desirable range. Be aware that the desired range may be different for some individuals due to their medical conditions, and what is desirable for one person may be considered high in another.

Table 8.3. Result Ranges for Lipoprotein Panel

Total Cholesterol Level	Total Cholesterol Category
Less than 200 mg/dL	Desirable
200–239 mg/dL	Borderline high
240 mg/dL and above	High

LDL Cholesterol Level	LDL Cholesterol Category
Less than 100 mg/dL	Optimal
100–129 mg/dL	Near optimal/above optimal
130–159 mg/dL	Borderline high
160–189 mg/dL	High
190 mg/dL and above	Very high

HDL Cholesterol Level	HDL Cholesterol Category
Less than 40 mg/dL	A major risk factor for heart disease
40–59 mg/dL	The higher, the better
60 mg/dL and above	Considered protective against heart disease

Note: mg/dL = milligrams per deciliter.

Adapted from "Common Blood Tests," National Heart, Lung, and Blood Institute (NHLBI, www.nhlbi.nih.gov), January 2010.

Chapter 9

EKG and Stress Tests

Understanding Electrocardiography

An electrocardiogram, or EKG, is a simple, painless test that re-cords the heart's electrical activity. To understand this test, it will help to briefly review how the heart's electrical system works. With each heartbeat, an electrical signal spreads from the top of the heart to the bottom. As it travels, the signal causes the heart to contract and pump blood. The process repeats with each new heartbeat. The heart's electrical signals set the rhythm of the heartbeat. See chap-ter 1 for more information about heart anatomy, and see chapter 4 for more details about the heart's electrical system.

An EKG shows how fast your heart is beating and whether the rhythm of your heartbeat is steady or irregular. It also shows the strength and timing of electrical signals as they pass through each part of your heart.

This test is used to detect and evaluate many heart problems, such as heart attack, arrhythmia, and heart failure. EKG results also can suggest other disorders that affect heart function.

EKGs also are used to monitor how the heart is working. This chapter focuses on how EKGs are used for testing purposes.

Other Names for an Electrocardiogram

An electrocardiogram also is called EKG or ECG. Sometimes the test is called a 12 lead EKG or 12 lead ECG because the electrical activity of the heart is most often recorded from 12 different places on the body at the same time.

When an EKG Is Necessary

Your doctor may recommend an EKG if you have signs or symptoms that suggest a heart problem. Examples of such signs and symptoms include chest pain; heart pounding, racing, or fluttering; and the sense your heart is beating unevenly. Problems breathing or feeling tired and weak can also be suggestive of a heart problem. If your doctor hears any unusual heart sounds when listening to your heartbeat, an EKG may be recommended. In addition, you may need to have more than one EKG so your doctor can diagnose certain heart conditions.

An EKG may be done as part of a routine health exam to screen for early heart disease without symptoms. However, many experts recommend against this because a normal EKG does not always mean the heart is healthy, and an abnormal EKG does not necessarily mean heart disease is present. Your doctor is more likely to look for early heart disease if your mother, father, brother, or sister had heart disease—especially if it developed early.

You may have an EKG so your doctor can check how well heart medicine or a medical device, such as a pacemaker, is working. The test also may be used for routine screening before major surgery.

Your doctor may use EKG results to help plan your treatment for a heart condition.

What to Expect before an EKG

No special preparation is needed for an EKG. Before the test, let your doctor or doctor's office know what medicines you're taking. Some medicines can affect EKG results.

What to Expect during an EKG

An EKG is painless and harmless. A technician attaches soft, sticky patches called electrodes to the skin of your chest, arms, and legs. The patches are about the size of a quarter.

Typically, 12 patches are attached to detect your heart's electrical activity from many angles. To help the patches stick, the technician may have to shave areas of your skin.

After the patches are placed on your skin, you lie still on a table while the patches detect your heart's electrical signals. A machine records these signals on graph paper or displays them on a screen.

The entire test takes about 10 minutes.

What to Expect after an EKG

After an EKG, the electrodes (soft patches) are removed from your skin. You may get a rash or redness where the EKG patches were attached. This mild rash usually goes away without treatment.

You usually can go back to your normal daily routine after an EKG.

Special Types of EKG

The standard EKG described above, called a resting 12 lead EKG, records only seconds of heart activity at a time. It will show a heart problem only if the problem is present during the time the test is run.

Many heart problems are present all the time, and a resting 12 lead EKG will detect them. But some heart problems, like those related to an irregular heartbeat, can come and go. They may occur for only a few minutes of the day or only while you exercise. Special

EKGs, such as stress tests and Holter and event monitors, are used to help diagnose these kinds of problems.

In addition, some heart problems are easier to diagnose when your heart is working hard and beating fast. During stress testing, you exercise to make your heart work hard and beat fast while your heart's electrical activity is recorded. If you're not able to exercise, you're given medicine to make your heart work hard and beat fast.

Stress testing is explained in greater detail later in this chapter. Holter and event monitors are discussed in chapter 10.

EKG Results

Many heart problems change the heart's electrical activity in distinct ways. An EKG can help detect a number of heart problems.

EKG recordings can help doctors diagnose a heart attack that's happening currently or has happened in the past. This is especially true if doctors can compare a current EKG recording to an older one. An EKG also can show the following things:

- Lack of blood flow to the heart muscle

- A heart that's beating too fast, too slow, or with an irregular rhythm (arrhythmia)

- A heart that doesn't pump forcefully enough (heart failure)

- Heart muscle that's too thick or parts of the heart that are too big

- Birth defects in the heart (congenital heart defects)

- Problems with the heart valves (heart valve disease)

- Inflammation of the sac that surrounds the heart (pericarditis)

An EKG also can reveal whether the heartbeat starts at the top right part of the heart like it should. The test shows how long it takes for the electrical signals to travel through the heart. Delays in signal travel time may suggest heart block or long QT syndrome.

EKG Risks

An EKG has no serious risks. It's a harmless, painless test that detects the heart's electrical activity. EKGs don't give off electrical charges, such as shocks. You may have a mild rash where the electrodes (soft patches) were attached. This rash usually goes away without treatment.

Understanding Stress Testing

Because some heart problems are easier to diagnose when your heart is working hard and beating fast, your doctor may order a stress test. Stress testing gives your doctor information about how your heart works during physical stress.

During a stress test, you exercise (walk or run on a treadmill or pedal a bicycle) to make your heart work hard and beat fast. Tests are done on your heart while you exercise. If you have arthritis or another medical problem that prevents you from exercising during a stress test, your doctor may give you medicine to make your heart work hard as if during exercise. This is called a pharmacological stress test.

Overview

Doctors usually use stress testing to help diagnose coronary heart disease (CHD). They also use stress testing to see how severe CHD is in people who are already known to have it.

You may not have any signs or symptoms of CHD when your heart is at rest. But when your heart has to work harder during exercise, it needs more blood and oxygen. Narrowed arteries can't supply enough blood for your heart to work well. As a result, signs and symptoms of CHD may occur only during exercise.

A stress test can detect problems, such as abnormal changes in your heart rate or blood pressure, which may suggest your heart isn't getting enough blood during exercise. It can also help determine whether symptoms such as shortness of breath or chest pain are related to a heart problem versus another cause. Stress testing can also identify any abnormal changes in your heart's rhythm or electrical activity.

During a stress test, if you can't exercise for as long as what's considered normal for someone your age, it may be a sign not enough blood is flowing to your heart. However, other factors besides CHD can prevent you from exercising long enough (for example, lung disease, anemia, or poor general fitness).

A stress test also may be used to assess other problems, such as heart valve disease or heart failure.

There are two main types of stress testing: a standard exercise stress test and an imaging stress test.

Standard Exercise Stress Test

A standard exercise stress test uses an EKG to detect and record the heart's electrical activity—how fast your heart is beating, the heart's rhythm, and the strength and timing of electrical signals as they pass through each part of your heart.

During a standard stress test, your blood pressure will be checked. You also may be asked to breathe into a special tube during the test. This allows your doctor to see how well you're breathing and measure the gases you breathe out.

A standard stress test shows changes in your heart's electrical activity. It also may show signs your heart isn't getting enough blood during exercise.

Imaging Stress Test

Some stress tests take pictures of your heart when you exercise and when you're at rest. These imaging stress tests can show how well blood is flowing in various parts of your heart and how well your heart squeezes out blood when it beats.

One type of imaging stress test involves echocardiography (echo), further discussed in chapter 11. This test uses sound waves to create a moving picture of your heart. An exercise stress echo can show how well your heart's chambers and valves are working when your heart is under stress.

The test can identify areas of poor blood flow to your heart, dead heart muscle tissue, and areas of the heart muscle wall that aren't contracting normally. These areas may have been damaged during a heart attack, or they may not be getting enough blood.

Other imaging stress tests use radioactive dye to create pictures of the blood flow to your heart. The dye is injected into your bloodstream before the pictures of your heart are taken. The pictures show how much of the dye has reached various parts of your heart during exercise and while you're at rest.

Tests that use radioactive dye include a thallium or sestamibi stress test and a positron emission tomography (PET) stress test. The amount of radiation in the dye is thought to be safe and not a danger to you or those around you. However, if you're pregnant, you shouldn't have this test because of risks it might pose to your unborn child.

Imaging stress tests tend to be more accurate at detecting CHD than standard (nonimaging) stress tests. Imaging stress tests also can predict the risk of a future heart attack or premature death.

An imaging stress test may be done first (as opposed to a standard exercise stress test) if any of the following are true:

- You can't exercise for enough time to get your heart working at its hardest (medical problems, such as arthritis or leg arteries clogged by plaque, may prevent you from exercising enough)

- You have abnormal heartbeats or other problems that would cause a standard exercise stress test to be inaccurate

- You have had a heart procedure in the past, such as a coronary artery bypass grafting or the placement of a stent in a coronary artery

Other Names for Stress Testing

- Exercise echocardiogram or exercise stress echo
- Exercise test
- Myocardial perfusion imaging
- Nuclear stress test
- PET stress test
- Pharmacological stress test
- Sestamibi stress test
- Stress EKG
- Thallium stress test
- Treadmill test

When Stress Testing Is Necessary

You may need stress testing if you've had chest pains, shortness of breath, or other symptoms of limited blood flow to your heart. Imaging stress tests, particularly, can show whether you have CHD or a heart valve problem.

If you've been diagnosed with CHD or recently had a heart attack, a stress test can show whether you can tolerate an exercise program. If you've had angioplasty with or without stents or coronary artery bypass grafting, a stress test can show how well the treatment relieves your CHD symptoms.

You also may need a stress test if, during exercise, you feel faint, get a rapid heartbeat or a fluttering feeling in your chest, or have other symptoms of an arrhythmia (an abnormal heartbeat).

If you don't have chest pain when you exercise but still get short of breath, you may need a stress test. The test can help show whether a heart problem, rather than a lung problem or being out of shape, is causing your breathing problems.

For such testing, you breathe into a special tube. This allows a technician to measure the gases you breathe out. Breathing into the special tube and checking the heart as part of a stress test also is done before a heart transplant to help assess whether you're a candidate for surgery.

Stress testing isn't used as a routine screening test for CHD. Usually you have to have symptoms of CHD before a doctor will recommend stress testing. However, some doctors may want to use a stress test to screen for CHD in patients with diabetes, which increases your risk for CHD. However, studies have shown that screening diabetic patients with stress tests does not improve risks of heart attack or death.

What to Expect before Stress Testing

Standard stress testing often is done in a doctor's office. Imaging stress testing usually is done at a hospital. Be sure to wear athletic or other shoes in which you can exercise comfortably. You may be asked to wear comfortable clothes, or you may be given a gown to wear during the test.

Your doctor may ask you not to eat or drink anything but water for a short time before the test. If you're diabetic, ask your doctor whether you need to adjust your medicines on the day of your test.

For some stress tests, you can't drink coffee or other caffeinated drinks for a day before the test. Certain over-the-counter or prescription medicines also may interfere with some stress tests. Discuss with your doctor whether you need to avoid certain drinks or food or change how you take your medicine before the test.

If you use an inhaler for asthma or other breathing problems, bring it to the test. Make sure you let the doctor know you use it.

What to Expect during Stress Testing

During all types of stress testing, a technician or nurse will always be with you to closely check your health status.

Before you start the stress part of a stress test, the technician or nurse will put sticky patches called electrodes on your skin and prepare you for the EKG part of the test as described earlier. The technician or nurse will put a blood pressure cuff on your arm to check your blood pressure during the stress test. (The cuff will feel tight on your arm when it expands every few minutes.) Also, you may be asked to breathe into a special tube so the gases you breathe out can be measured.

After these preparations, you'll exercise on a treadmill or stationary bicycle. If such exercise poses a problem for you, you may instead turn a crank with your arms. During the test, the exercise level will get harder. You can stop whenever you feel the exercise is too much for you.

If you can't exercise, medicine may be injected into a vein in your arm or hand. This medicine will increase blood flow through your coronary arteries and make your heart beat fast, as would exercise. The stress test can then be done.

The medicine may make you flushed and anxious, but the effects go away as soon as the test is over. The medicine also may give you a headache.

While you're exercising or receiving medicine to make your heart work harder, the technician will frequently ask you how you're feeling. You should tell him or her if you feel chest pain, short of breath, or dizzy.

The exercise or medicine infusion will continue until you reach a target heart rate or until one or more of the following are true:

- You feel moderate to severe chest pain.

- You get too out of breath to continue.

- You develop abnormally high or low blood pressure or an arrhythmia (an abnormal heartbeat).

- You become dizzy.

The technician will continue to check your heart functions and blood pressure after the test until they return to your normal levels.

The stress part of a stress test (when you're exercising or receiving medicine that makes your heart work hard) usually lasts about 15 minutes or less. However, prep time before the test and monitoring time afterward extend the total test time to about an hour for a standard stress test and up to three hours or more for some imaging stress tests.

Exercise Stress Echocardiogram Test

For an exercise stress echocardiogram (echo) test, the technician will take pictures of your heart using echocardiography before you exercise and as soon as you finish.

A sonographer (a person who specializes in using ultrasound techniques) will apply gel to your chest. Then, he or she will briefly put a transducer (a wand-like device) against your chest and move it around. The transducer sends and receives high-pitched sounds you usually can't hear. The echoes from the sound waves are converted into moving pictures of your heart on a screen.

You may be asked to lie on your side on an exam table for this test. Some stress echo tests also use a dye to improve imaging. This dye is injected into your bloodstream during the test.

Sestamibi or Other Imaging Stress Tests Involving Radioactive Dye

For a sestamibi stress test, or other imaging stress tests that use radioactive dye, the technician will inject a small amount of dye (such as sestamibi) into your bloodstream. This is done through a needle placed in a vein in your arm or hand.

You're usually given the dye about a half hour before you start exercising or take medicine to make your heart work hard. The amount of radiation in the dye is thought to be safe and not a danger to you or those around you. However, if you're pregnant, you shouldn't have this test because of risks it might pose to your unborn child.

Pictures will be taken of your heart at least two times: when it's at rest and when it's working its hardest. You'll lie down on a table and a special camera or scanner that can see the dye in your bloodstream will take pictures of your heart.

Some pictures may not be taken until you lie quietly for a few hours after the stress test. Some patients may even be asked to return in a day or so for more pictures.

What to Expect after Stress Testing

After stress testing, you'll be able to return to your normal activities. If you had a test that involved radioactive dye, your doctor may ask you to drink plenty of fluids to flush it out of your body. You also shouldn't have certain other imaging tests until the dye is no longer in your body. Your doctor can advise you about this.

Stress Testing Risks

There's little risk of serious harm from any type of stress testing. The chance of these tests causing a heart attack or death is about one in 5,000. More common, but less serious, side effects linked to stress testing include the following:

- **Arrhythmia (an abnormal heartbeat):** Often, an arrhythmia will go away quickly once you're at rest. But if it persists, you may need monitoring or treatment in a hospital.

- **Low blood pressure, which can cause you to feel dizzy or faint:** This problem may go away once your heart stops working hard; it usually doesn't require treatment.

- **Jitteriness or discomfort while getting medicine to make your heart work harder (you may be given medicine if you can't exercise):** These side effects usually go away shortly after you stop getting the medicine. In some cases, the symptoms may last a few hours.

Also, some medicines used for pharmacological stress tests can cause wheezing, shortness of breath, and other asthma-like symptoms. In some cases, these symptoms may be severe and require treatment.

Stress Testing Results

Stress testing gives your doctor information about how your heart works during physical stress (exercise) and how healthy your heart is. Abnormal test results may be due to CHD or other factors, such as a lack of physical fitness.

If you have a standard exercise stress test and the results are normal, no further testing or treatment may be needed. But if your test results are abnormal, or if you're physically unable to exercise, your doctor may want you to have an imaging stress test or other tests.

Even if your standard exercise stress test results are normal, your doctor may want you to have an imaging stress test if you continue having symptoms (such as shortness of breath or chest pain). Imaging stress tests are more accurate than standard exercise stress tests, but they're much more expensive.

Imaging stress tests show how well blood is flowing in the heart muscle and reveal parts of the heart that aren't contracting strongly. They also can show the parts of the heart that aren't getting enough blood, as well as dead tissue in the heart, where no blood flows. (A heart attack can cause some tissue in the heart to die.)

If your imaging stress test suggests significant CHD, your doctor may want you to have more testing or treatment.

Adapted from "Electrocardiogram," November 2008, and "Stress Testing," June 2009, both produced by the National Heart, Lung, and Blood Institute (NHLBI, www.nhlbi.nih.gov).

Chapter 10

Holter and Event Monitors

Holter and event monitors are medical devices that record the heart's electrical activity. Doctors most often use these monitors to diagnose arrhythmias—problems with the speed or rhythm of the heartbeat.

Holter and event monitors also are used to detect silent myocardial ischemia. In this condition, not enough oxygen-rich blood reaches the heart muscle. Silent means no symptoms occur.

These monitors also can check whether treatments for arrhythmia and silent myocardial ischemia are working. This chapter focuses on using Holter and event monitors to diagnose problems with the heart's rate or rhythm.

Holter and event monitors are similar to an EKG. An EKG, as described in chapter 9, is a simple test that detects and records the heart's electrical activity. It's the most common test for diagnosing a heart rhythm problem. However, a standard EKG records the heartbeat for only a few seconds. It won't detect heart rhythm problems that don't occur during the test.

Holter and event monitors are small, portable devices. You can wear one while you do your normal daily activities, allowing the monitor to record your heart for a longer time than an EKG.

Some people have heart rhythm problems that occur only during certain activities, such as sleep or physical exertion. Using a Holter or event monitor increases the chance of recording these problems.

Although similar, Holter and event monitors aren't the same. A Holter monitor records your heart's electrical activity the entire time you're wearing it. An event monitor records your heart's electrical activity only at certain times while you're wearing it.

Types of Holter and Event Monitors

Holter Monitors

Holter monitors are sometimes called continuous EKGs because Holter monitors record your heart rhythm continuously for 24 to 48 hours.

A Holter monitor is about the size of a large deck of cards. You can clip it to a belt or carry it in a pocket. Wires connect the device to sensors (called electrodes) that are stuck to your chest using sticky patches. These sensors detect your heart's electrical signals, and the monitor records your heart's rhythm.

Wireless Holter Monitors

Wireless Holter monitors have a longer recording time than standard Holter monitors. Wireless monitors record your heart's electrical activity for a preset amount of time.

These monitors use wireless cellular technology to send the recorded data to your doctor's office or a company that checks the data. This happens automatically at certain times. Wireless monitors still have wires that connect the device to the sensors stuck to your chest.

You can use a wireless Holter monitor for days or even weeks until signs or symptoms of a heart rhythm problem occur. These monitors usually are used to detect heart rhythm problems that don't occur often.

Although wireless Holter monitors work for longer periods, they have a down side. You must remember to write down the time symptoms occur so your doctor can match it to the heart rhythm recording. Also, the batteries in the wireless monitor must be changed every one to two days.

Event Monitors

Event monitors are similar to Holter monitors. You wear one while you do your normal daily activities. Most event monitors have wires that connect the device to sensors. The sensors are stuck to your chest using sticky patches.

Unlike Holter monitors, event monitors don't continuously record your heart's electrical activity. They record only when symptoms occur. For many event monitors, you need to start the monitor when you feel symptoms. Some event monitors start automatically if they detect abnormal heart rhythms.

Event monitors tend to be smaller than Holter monitors because they don't need to store as much data.

Different types of event monitors work in slightly different ways. Your doctor will explain how to use the monitor before you start wearing it.

Postevent Recorders

Postevent recorders are among the smallest event monitors. You can wear a postevent recorder like a wristwatch or carry it in your pocket. The pocket version is about the size of a thick credit card. These monitors don't have wires to connect the device to chest sensors.

When you feel a symptom, you start the recorder. A postevent recorder records only what happens after you start it. It may miss a heart rhythm problem that occurs before and during the onset of symptoms. Also, it may be hard to start the monitor when a symptom is in progress.

In some cases, this missing data could have helped your doctor diagnose the heart rhythm problem.

Presymptom Memory Loop Recorders

Presymptom memory loop recorders are the size of a small cell phone. They're also called continuous loop event recorders.

You can clip this event monitor to your belt or carry it in your pocket. Wires connect the device to sensors on your chest.

These recorders are always recording and erasing data. When you feel a symptom, you push a button on the device. The normal erase process stops. The recording will show a few minutes of data from before, during, and after the symptom. This may make it possible for your doctor to see very brief changes in your heart rhythm.

Autodetect Recorders

Autodetect recorders are about the size of the palm of your hand. Wires connect the device to sensors on your chest.

You don't need to start an autodetect recorder during symptoms. These recorders detect abnormal heart rhythms and automatically record and send the data to your doctor's office.

Implantable Loop Recorders

You may need an implantable loop recorder if other event monitors can't provide enough data. Implantable loop recorders are about the size of a pack of gum. This type of event monitor is inserted under the skin on your chest. No wires or chest sensors are used.

Your doctor can program the device to record when you start it during symptoms or automatically if it detects an abnormal heart rhythm. Devices may differ, so your doctor will tell you how to use your recorder. In some cases, a special card is held close to the recorder to start it.

Other Names for Holter and Event Monitors

Various Holter and event monitors are known by several different names:

- Ambulatory EKG or ECG
- Episodic monitors
- Mobile cardiac outpatient telemetry systems (this is another name for autodetect recorders)
- Transtelephonic event monitors (these monitors require the patient to send the collected data by telephone to a doctor's office or a company that checks the data)

When a Holter or Event Monitor Is Necessary

Holter and event monitors most often are used to detect arrhythmias in people who have had the following problems:

- **Fainting or sometimes feeling dizzy:** A monitor may be used if causes other than a heart rhythm problem have been ruled out.

- **Palpitations that recur with no known cause:** Palpitations are feelings that your heart is skipping a beat, fluttering, or beating too hard or fast. You may have these feelings in your chest, throat, or neck.

People who are being treated for heart rhythm problems also may need to use Holter or event monitors. The monitors can show how treatments are working.

Heart rhythm problems may occur only at certain times, such as during sleep or physical exertion. Holter and event monitors record your heart rhythm while you do your normal daily routine. This allows your doctor to see how your heart responds to different daily activities, which can help diagnose the problem.

What to Expect before Using a Holter or Event Monitor

Your doctor will do a physical exam before giving you a Holter or event monitor. He or she will do the following things:

- Check your pulse to find out how fast your heart is beating (your heart rate) and whether your heart rhythm is steady or irregular

- Measure your blood pressure

- Check for swelling in your legs or feet; swelling could be a sign of an enlarged heart or heart failure, which could cause an arrhythmia

- Look for signs of other diseases that could be causing heart rhythm problems, such as thyroid disease

You may have an EKG test before your doctor sends you home with a Holter or event monitor. Your doctor will explain how to wear and use the Holter or event monitor. Usually you'll leave the office wearing it.

What to Expect while Using a Holter or Event Monitor

Your experience while using a Holter or event monitor depends on the type of monitor you have. However, most monitors have some factors in common.

Recording the Heart's Electrical Activity

All monitors record the heart's electrical activity, so it's important to maintain a clear signal between the sensors (electrodes) and the recording device.

In most cases, the sensors are attached to your chest with sticky patches. Wires connect the sensors to the monitor. You usually can clip the monitor to your belt or carry it in your pocket. (Postevent and implantable loop recorders don't have chest sensors.)

A good connection between the patches and your skin helps provide a clear signal. Poor contact leads to a poor recording that's hard for your doctor to read.

Oil, too much sweat, and hair can keep the patches from sticking to your skin. You may need to shave the area on your chest where your doctor will attach the patches. If you have to replace the patches, you'll need to clean the area with a special prep pad the doctor will provide.

You may need to use a small amount of special paste or gel to help the patches stick to your skin. Some patches come with paste or gel on them.

Too much movement can pull the patches away from your skin or create noise on the EKG strip. An EKG strip is a graph showing the pattern of your heartbeat. Noise looks like a lot of jagged lines; it makes it hard for your doctor to see the real rhythm of your heart.

When you have a symptom, stop what you're doing. This will ensure the recording shows your heart's activity rather than your movement.

Your doctor will tell you whether you need to adjust your activity level during the testing period. If you exercise, choose a cool location to avoid sweating too much. This will help the patches stay sticky.

Other everyday items also can disrupt the signal between the sensors and the monitor. These items include magnets, metal detectors, microwave ovens, and electric blankets, toothbrushes, and razors. Avoid using these items. Also avoid areas with high voltage.

Cell phones and MP3 players (such as iPods) may interfere with the signal if they're too close to the monitor. When using any electronic device, try to keep it at least 6 inches away from the monitor.

Keeping a Diary

When using a Holter or event monitor, you need to keep a diary of your symptoms and activities. Write down when symptoms occur, what they are, and what you were doing at the time.

It's important to note the time symptoms occur because your doctor matches the data with the information in your diary. This allows your doctor to see whether certain activities trigger changes in your heart rate and rhythm.

You also should include details in your diary about when you take any medicine or if you feel stress at certain times during the testing period.

What to Expect with Specific Monitors

Holter Monitors

You'll wear a Holter monitor for 24 to 48 hours. You can't get your monitor wet, so you won't be able to bathe or shower. You can take a sponge bath if needed.

When the testing period is complete, you'll return the device to your doctor's office. The results will be stored on the device.

The recording period for a standard Holter monitor may be too short to capture a heart rhythm problem. If this is the case, your doctor may recommend a wireless Holter monitor.

Wireless Holter Monitors

Wireless monitors record for a preset amount of time. Then they automatically send data to your doctor's office or a company that checks the data. These monitors use wireless cellular technology to send their data. However, they still have wires that connect the device to the sensors stuck to your chest.

You can use a wireless Holter monitor for days or even weeks until signs or symptoms of a heart rhythm problem occur. The batteries in the wireless monitor must be changed every one to two days. You'll need to detach the sensors to shower or bathe and then reattach them.

Event Monitors

Event monitors are slightly smaller than Holter monitors. They can be worn for weeks or until symptoms occur. Most event monitors are worn like Holter monitors—clipped to a belt or carried in a pocket. When you have symptoms, you simply push a button on your monitor to start recording. Some event monitors start automatically if they detect abnormal heart rhythms.

Postevent Recorders

Postevent recorders may be worn like a wristwatch or carried in a pocket. The pocket version is about the size of a thick credit card. These recorders don't have wires that connect the device to chest sensors.

To start the recorder when you feel a symptom, you hold it to your chest. To start the wristwatch version, you touch a button on the side of the watch.

You send the stored data to your doctor's office using a telephone. Your doctor will explain how to use the monitor before you leave his or her office.

Autodetect Recorders

Autodetect recorders are about the size of the palm of your hand. Wires connect the device to sensors on your chest.

You don't need to start an autodetect recorder. This type of monitor automatically starts recording if it detects abnormal heart rhythms. It then sends the data to your doctor's office.

Implantable Loop Recorders

Implantable loop recorders are about the size of a pack of gum. This type of event monitor is inserted under the skin on your chest. Your doctor will discuss the procedure with you. No chest sensors are used for implantable loop recorders.

Your doctor can program the device to record when you start it during symptoms or automatically if it detects an abnormal heart rhythm. Devices may differ, so your doctor will tell you how to use your recorder. In some cases, a special card is held close to the recorder to start it.

What to Expect after Using a Holter or Event Monitor

After you're finished using a Holter or event monitor, you'll return it to your doctor's office or the place where you picked it up.

If you were using an implantable loop recorder, it will need to be removed from your chest. Your doctor will discuss the procedure with you.

Your doctor will tell you when to expect the results. Once your doctor has reviewed the recordings, he or she will discuss the results with you.

Holter or Event Monitor Risks

The sticky patches used to attach the sensors (electrodes) to your chest have a small risk of skin irritation. You also may have an allergic reaction to the paste or gel that's sometimes used to attach the patches. The irritation will go away once the patches are removed.

If you're using an implantable loop recorder, you may get an infection or have pain where the device is placed under the skin. Your doctor may prescribe medicine to treat these problems.

Holter and event monitors have few risks.

Holter or Event Monitor Results

A Holter or event monitor may show what's causing the symptoms of an arrhythmia. A Holter or event monitor also can show whether a heart rhythm problem is harmless or requires treatment. The monitor may alert your doctor to medical conditions that can result in heart failure, stroke, or sudden cardiac arrest.

If the symptoms of a heart rhythm problem occur often, a Holter or event monitor has a good chance of capturing them. You may not have symptoms while using a monitor. Even so, your doctor may learn more about your heart rhythm from the test results.

Sometimes, Holter and event monitors can't help doctors diagnose heart rhythm problems. If this happens, talk with your doctor about other steps you can take.

One option may be to try a different type of monitor. Wireless Holter monitors and implantable loop recorders have longer recording periods. This may allow the monitor to get the data your doctor needs to make a diagnosis.

Adapted from "Holter and Event Monitors," National Heart, Lung, and Blood Institute (NHLBI, www.nhlbi.nih.gov), February 2010.

Chapter 11

Echocardiographs

Understanding Echocardiography

Echocardiography, or echo, is a painless test that uses sound waves to create pictures of your heart.

The test gives your doctor information about the size and shape of your heart and how well your heart's chambers and valves are working. Echo also can be done to detect heart problems in infants and children.

The test also can identify areas of heart muscle that aren't contracting normally due to poor blood flow or injury from a previous heart attack. In addition, a type of echo called Doppler ultrasound shows how well blood flows through the chambers and valves of your heart.

Echo can detect possible blood clots inside the heart, fluid buildup in the pericardium (the sac around the heart), and problems with the aorta. The aorta is the main artery that carries oxygen-rich blood from your heart to your body.

When Echocardiography Is Necessary

Your doctor may recommend echocardiography if you have signs and symptoms of heart problems. For example, shortness of breath and swelling in the legs can be due to weakness of the heart (heart failure), which can be seen on an echocardiogram.

Your doctor also may use echo to learn about the following things:

- **The size of your heart:** An enlarged heart can be the result of high blood pressure, leaky heart valves, or heart failure.

- **Heart muscles that are weak and aren't moving (pumping) properly:** Weakened areas of heart muscle can be due to damage from a heart attack. Weakening also can mean the area isn't getting enough blood supply, which may be due to coronary heart disease (also called coronary artery disease).

- **Problems with your heart valves:** Echo can show whether any of your heart valves don't open normally or don't form a complete seal when closed.

- **Problems with your heart's structure:** Echo can detect many structural problems, such as a hole in the septum or other congenital heart defects. The septum is the wall that separates the two chambers on the left side of the heart from the two chambers on the right side. Congenital heart defects are structural problems present at birth. Infants and children may have echo to detect these heart defects.

- **Blood clots or tumors:** If you've had a stroke, echo might be done to check for blood clots or tumors that may have caused it.

Your doctor also may use echo to see how well your heart responds to certain heart treatments, such as those used for heart failure.

Types of Echocardiography

There are several types of echocardiography. All use sound waves to create pictures of your heart. This is the same technology that allows doctors to see an unborn baby inside a pregnant woman.

Unlike x-rays and some other tests, echo doesn't involve radiation.

Transthoracic Echo

Transthoracic echo is the most common type of echocardiogram test. It's painless and noninvasive. Noninvasive means no surgery is done and no instruments are inserted into your body.

This type of echo involves placing a device called a transducer on your chest. The device sends special sound waves, called ultrasound, through your chest wall to your heart. The human ear can't hear ultrasound waves.

As the ultrasound waves bounce off the structures of your heart, a computer in the echo machine converts them into pictures on a screen.

Stress Echo

Stress echo is done as part of a stress test. During a stress test, you exercise or take medicine (given by your doctor) to make your heart work hard and beat fast. A technician will take pictures of your heart using echo before you exercise and as soon as you finish. This type of test is discussed in chapter 9, "EKG and Stress Tests."

Transesophageal Echo

With standard transthoracic echo, it can be hard to see the aorta and other parts of your heart. If your doctor needs a better look at these areas, he or she may recommend transesophageal echo (TEE). During this test, the transducer is attached to the end of a flexible tube. The tube is guided down your throat and into your esophagus (the passage leading from your mouth to your stomach). This allows your doctor to get more detailed pictures of your heart.

Fetal Echo

Fetal echo is used to look at an unborn baby's heart. A doctor may recommend this test to check a baby for heart problems. Fetal echo is commonly done during pregnancy at about 18 to 22 weeks. For this test, the transducer is moved over the pregnant woman's belly.

Three-Dimensional Echo

A three-dimensional (3D) echo creates 3D images of your heart. These images provide more information about how your heart looks and works. During transthoracic echo or transesophageal echo, 3D images can be taken as part of the process for these types of echo.

Three-dimensional echo may be used to diagnose heart problems in children. This method also may be used for planning and monitoring heart valve surgery.

Researchers continue to study new ways to use 3D echo.

What to Expect before Echocardiography

Echocardiography is done in a doctor's office or a hospital. No special preparations are needed for most types of echo. Usually you can eat, drink, and take any medicines as normal.

The exception is if you're having a transesophageal echo. This test usually requires that you don't eat or drink for eight hours prior to the test.

If you're having a stress echo, there may be special preparations. Your doctor will let you know how to prepare for your echo test.

What to Expect during Echocardiography

Echocardiography is painless and usually takes less than an hour. For some types of echo, your doctor will need to inject saline or a special dye into one of your veins to make your heart show up more clearly on the test images. This special dye is different from the dye used during angiography (a test used to examine the body's blood vessels).

For most types of echo, you'll be asked to remove your clothing from the waist up. Women will be given a gown to wear during the test. You'll lie on your back or left side on an exam table or stretcher.

Soft, sticky patches called electrodes will be attached to your chest to allow an EKG to be done. An EKG is a test that records the heart's electrical activity.

A doctor or sonographer (a person specially trained to do ultra-sounds) will apply gel to your chest. The gel helps the sound waves reach your heart. A wand-like device called a transducer will then be moved around on your chest.

The transducer transmits ultrasound waves into your chest. Echoes from the sound waves will be converted into pictures of your heart on a computer screen. During the test, the lights in the room will be dimmed so the computer screen is easier to see.

The sonographer will make several recordings of the pictures to show various locations in your heart. The recordings will be put on a computer disc or videotape for the cardiologist (heart specialist) to review.

During the test, you may be asked to change positions or hold your breath for a short time so the sonographer can get good pictures of your heart.

At times, the sonographer may apply a bit of pressure to your chest with the transducer. This pressure can be a little uncomfortable, but it helps get the best picture of your heart. You should let the sonographer know if you feel too uncomfortable.

This process is similar for fetal echo. However, in that test the transducer is placed over the pregnant woman's belly at the location of the baby's heart.

Transesophageal Echo

TEE is used when your doctor needs a more detailed view of your heart. For example, TEE may be used to look for blood clots in your heart. A doctor, not a sonographer, performs this type of echo.

The test uses the same technology as transthoracic echo, but the transducer is attached to the end of a flexible tube. The tube will be guided down your throat and into your esophagus (the passage leading from your mouth to your stomach). From this angle, your doctor can get a more detailed image of your heart and the major blood vessels leading to and from your heart.

For TEE, you'll likely be given medicine to help you relax during the test. The medicine will be injected into one of your veins. Your blood pressure, the oxygen content of your blood, and other vital signs will be checked during the test. You'll be given oxygen through a tube in your nose. If you wear dentures or partials, you'll have to remove them.

The back of your mouth will be numbed with a gel or a spray so you don't gag when the transducer is put down your throat. The tube with the transducer on the end will be gently placed in your throat and guided down until it's in place behind the heart.

The pictures of your heart are then recorded as your doctor moves the transducer around in your esophagus and stomach. You shouldn't feel any discomfort as this happens.

Although the imaging usually takes less than an hour, you may be watched for a few hours at the doctor's office or hospital after the test.

Stress Echo

Stress echo is a transthoracic echo combined with either an exercise or pharmacological stress test. For an exercise stress test, you'll walk or run on a treadmill or pedal a stationary bike to make your heart work hard and beat fast. For a pharmacological stress test, you'll be given medicine to make your heart work hard and beat fast. A technician will take pictures of your heart using echo before you exercise and as soon as you finish.

What You May See and Hear during Echocardiography

As the doctor or sonographer moves the transducer around, different views of your heart can be seen on the screen of the echo machine. The structures of the heart will appear as white objects, while any fluid or blood will appear black on the screen.

Doppler ultrasound techniques often are used during echo tests. Doppler ultrasound is a special ultrasound that shows how blood is flowing through the blood vessels.

This test allows the sonographer to see blood flowing at different speeds and in different directions. The speeds and directions appear as different colors moving within the black and white images.

The human ear is unable to hear the sound waves used in echo. If Doppler ultrasound is used, you may be able to hear whooshing sounds. Your doctor can use these sounds to learn about blood flow through your heart.

What to Expect after Echocardiography

You usually can go back to your normal activities right after having echocardiography, although if you have a TEE, you may be watched for a few hours at the doctor's office or hospital after the test. Your throat might be sore for a few hours after the test. You also may not be able to drive right after a TEE. Your doctor will let you know whether you need to arrange for someone to take you home.

Echocardiography Risks

Transthoracic and fetal echocardiography have no risks. These tests are safe in adults, children, and infants.

If you have a TEE, some risks are associated with the medicine given to help you relax. These include a reaction to the medicine, problems breathing, or nausea (feeling sick to your stomach). Your throat also might be sore for a few hours after the test. Rarely, the tube used during TEE can cause minor throat injuries.

Stress echo has some risks, but they're related to the exercise or medicine used to raise your heart rate, not to the echo. Serious complications from stress tests are very uncommon.

Echocardiography Results

Echo can detect many heart problems. Some may be minor and pose no risk to you. Others can be signs of serious heart disease or other heart conditions.

Echocardiography shows the size, structure, and movement of the various parts of your heart, including the valves, the septum (the wall separating the right and left heart chambers), and the walls of the heart chambers. Doppler ultrasound shows the movement of blood through the heart. Echo can be used to diagnose heart problems, guide or determine next steps for treatment, monitor changes and improvement, or determine the need for more tests.

Adapted from "Echocardiography," National Heart, Lung, and Blood Institute (NHLBI, www.nhlbi.nih.gov), August 2009.

Chapter 12

Nuclear Heart Scans

Understanding Nuclear Heart Scanning

A nuclear heart scan is a test that allows your doctor to get important information about the health of your heart. During a nuclear heart scan, a safe, radioactive substance called a tracer is injected into your bloodstream through a vein. The tracer travels to your heart and releases energy. Special cameras outside your body detect the energy and use it to create pictures of your heart.

Nuclear heart scans are used for three main purposes:

- **To check how blood is flowing to the heart muscle:** If part of the heart muscle isn't getting blood, it may be a sign of coronary heart disease (CHD), also called coronary artery disease. CHD can lead to angina, heart attack, and other heart problems. When a nuclear heart scan is done for this purpose, it's called myocardial perfusion scanning.

- **To look for damaged heart muscle:** Damage may be the result of a previous heart attack, injury, infection, or medicine. When a nuclear heart scan is done for this purpose, it's called myocardial viability testing.

- **To see how well your heart pumps blood to your body:** When a nuclear heart scan is done for this purpose, it's called ventricular function scanning.

Usually, two sets of pictures are taken during a nuclear heart scan. The first set is taken right after a stress test, while your heart is beating fast.

During a stress test, you exercise to make your heart work hard and beat fast. If you can't exercise, you may be given medicine to increase your heart rate. This is called a pharmacological stress test.

The second set of pictures is taken later, while your heart is at rest and beating at a normal rate.

Types of Nuclear Heart Scanning

The two main types of nuclear heart scanning are single positron emission computed tomography (SPECT) and cardiac positron emission tomography (PET).

SPECT is the most well established and widely used type, while PET is newer. There are specific reasons for using each.

Single Positron Emission Computed Tomography

SPECT is the most common nuclear scanning test for diagnosing CHD. Combining SPECT with a stress test can show problems with blood flow to the heart that can be detected only when the heart is working hard and beating fast.

SPECT also is used to look for areas of damaged or dead heart muscle tissue. These areas may be the result of a previous heart attack or other cause.

SPECT also can show how well the heart's lower left chamber (left ventricle) pumps blood to the body. Weak pumping ability may be the result of a heart attack, heart failure, and other causes.

The most commonly used tracers in SPECT are called thallium-201, technetium-99m sestamibi (Cardiolite®), and technetium-99m tetrofosmin (Myoview™).

Positron Emission Tomography

PET uses different tracers than SPECT. PET can provide more detailed pictures of the heart. However, PET is newer and has some technical limits that make it less available than SPECT.

Research into advances in both SPECT and PET is ongoing. Right now, there's no clear-cut advantage to using one over the other in all situations.

PET can be used for the same purposes as SPECT—to diagnose CHD, check for damaged or dead heart muscle tissue, and check the heart's pumping strength.

PET takes a clearer picture through thick layers of tissue (such as abdominal or breast tissue). PET also is better than SPECT at showing whether CHD is affecting more than one of your heart's blood vessels.

A PET scan also may be used if a SPECT scan doesn't produce good pictures.

What to Expect before a Nuclear Heart Scan

A nuclear heart scan can take a lot of time. Most scans take between two and five hours, especially if two sets of pictures are needed.

Discuss with your doctor how a nuclear heart scan is done. Talk with him or her about your overall health, including health problems such as asthma, chronic obstructive pulmonary disease (COPD), diabetes, and kidney disease.

If you have lung disease or diabetes, your doctor will give you special instructions before the nuclear heart scan.

If you're having a stress test as part of your nuclear heart scan, wear comfortable walking shoes and loose-fitting clothes for the test. You may be asked to wear a hospital gown during the test.

Let your doctor know about any medicines you take, including prescription and over-the-counter medicines, vitamins, minerals, and other supplements. Some medicines and supplements can interfere with the medicines that may be used during the stress test to increase your heart rate.

What to Expect during a Nuclear Heart Scan

Many, but not all, nuclear medicine centers are located in hospitals. A doctor who has special training in nuclear heart scans—a cardiologist or radiologist—will oversee the test. Cardiologists are doctors who specialize in diagnosing and treating heart problems. Radiologists are doctors who specialize in diagnostic techniques, such as nuclear scans.

Before the test begins, the doctor or a technician will use a needle to insert an intravenous (IV) line into a vein in your arm. Through this IV line, he or she will put the radioactive tracer into your bloodstream at the right time. You also will have EKG patches attached to your body to check your heart rate during the test.

During the Stress Test

If you're having an exercise stress test as part of your nuclear scan, you'll walk on a treadmill or pedal a stationary bicycle. You'll be attached to EKG and blood pressure monitors.

You'll be asked to exercise until you're too tired to continue, short of breath, or having chest or leg pain. You can expect your heart will beat faster, you'll breathe faster, your blood pressure will increase, and you'll sweat.

Tell the doctor if you have any chest, arm, or jaw pain or discomfort. Also report any dizziness, light-headedness, or other unusual symptoms.

If you're unable to exercise, your doctor may give you medicine to make your heart beat faster. This is called a pharmacological stress test. The medicine may make you feel anxious, sick, dizzy, or shaky for a short time. If the side effects are severe, your doctor may give you other medicine for relief.

Before the exercise or pharmacological stress test stops, the tracer is injected through the IV line.

During the Nuclear Heart Scan

The nuclear heart scan will start shortly after the stress test. You'll lie very still on a padded table.

The nuclear heart scan camera, called a gamma camera, is enclosed in a metal housing. The part of the camera that detects the tracer's radioactivity can be put in several positions around your body as you lie on the padded table.

For some nuclear heart scans, the metal housing is shaped like a doughnut and you lie on a table that moves slowly through the doughnut hole. The computer used to collect the pictures of your heart is nearby or in another room.

Usually, two sets of pictures are taken. One will be taken right after the stress test and the other will be taken after a period of rest. The pictures may be taken all in one day or over two days. It takes about 15 to 30 minutes to take each set of pictures.

Some people find it hard to stay in one position for some time. Others may feel anxious while lying in the doughnut-shaped scanner. The table may feel hard. Sometimes the room may feel chilly because of the air conditioning needed to maintain the machines.

Let the doctor or technician know how you're feeling during the test so he or she can respond as needed.

What to Expect after a Nuclear Heart Scan

Your doctor may ask you to return to the nuclear medicine center on a second day for more pictures. Outpatients will be allowed to go home after the scan or leave the nuclear medicine center between the two scans.

Most people can go back to their daily activities after a nuclear heart scan. The radioactivity will naturally leave your body in your urine or stool. It's helpful to drink plenty of fluids after the test.

The cardiologist or radiologist will read and interpret the results of the test within one to three days. Results will be reported to your doctor, who will contact you to discuss them, or the cardiologist or radiologist may discuss the results directly with you.

Nuclear Heart Scan Risks

The radioactive tracer used during a nuclear heart scan exposes the body to a very small amount of radiation. No long-term effects have been reported from these doses.

Radiation dose might be a concern for people who need multiple scans. However, advances in hardware and software may greatly reduce the radiation dose people receive.

Some people are allergic to the radioactive tracer, but this is very rare.

If you have CHD, you may have chest pain during the stress test when you exercise or are given medicine to increase your heart rate. Medicine can relieve this symptom.

If you're pregnant, tell your doctor or technician before the scan. The test may be postponed until after your pregnancy.

Nuclear Heart Scan Results

The results from a nuclear heart scan can help doctors do the following things:

- Diagnose heart conditions, such as CHD, and decide the best course of treatment

- Manage certain heart diseases, such as CHD and heart failure, and predict short-term or long-term survival

- Determine your risk for a heart attack

- Decide whether other heart tests or procedures will help you; examples of these tests and procedures include coronary angiography and cardiac catheterization

- Decide whether procedures that can increase blood flow to the coronary arteries will help you; examples of these procedures include angioplasty and coronary artery bypass grafting (CABG)

- Monitor procedures or surgeries that have been done, such as CABG or a heart transplant

Adapted from "Nuclear Heart Scan," National Heart, Lung, and Blood Institute (NHLBI, www.nhlbi.nih.gov), January 2010.

Chapter 13

Cardiac CT
Scans and MRIs

Cardiac Computed Tomography

Cardiac computed tomography, or cardiac CT, is a painless test that uses an x-ray machine to take clear, detailed pictures of the heart. During a cardiac CT scan, an x-ray machine will move around your body in a circle. The machine will take a picture of each part of your heart. A computer will put the pictures together to make a 3D picture of the whole heart. This picture shows the inside of the heart and the structures that surround the heart. This common test is used to look for problems in the heart.

In most cases, an iodine-based dye (contrast dye) is injected into one of your veins during the scan. The contrast dye travels through your blood vessels, which helps highlight them on the x-ray pictures.

What to Expect before Cardiac CT

Your doctor will tell you how to prepare for the cardiac CT scan. People usually are asked to avoid drinks that contain caffeine before the test. Normally you're allowed to drink water, but you're asked not to eat for four hours before the scan.

If you take medicine for diabetes, talk with your doctor about whether you'll need to change how you take it on the day of your cardiac CT scan.

Tell your doctor if you are pregnant or may be pregnant. Even though cardiac CT uses a low radiation dose, you shouldn't have the scan if you're pregnant. The x-rays may harm the fetus. Also tell your doctor if you have asthma or kidney problems or are allergic to any medicines, iodine, or shellfish. These problems may increase your chance of having an allergic reaction to the contrast dye sometimes used during cardiac CT.

A technician will ask you to remove your clothes above the waist and wear a hospital gown. You also will be asked to remove any jewelry from around your neck or chest.

Taking pictures of the heart can be hard because the heart is always beating (in motion). A slower heart rate will help produce better quality pictures.

If you don't have asthma, COPD, or heart failure, your doctor may give you a medicine called a beta blocker to help slow your heart rate. The medicine will be given by mouth or injected into a vein.

What to Expect during Cardiac CT

The cardiac CT scan will take place in a hospital or outpatient office. A doctor who has experience with CT scanning will supervise the test.

Your doctor may want to use an iodine-based dye (contrast dye) during the cardiac CT scan. If so, a needle connected to an IV line will be put in a vein in your hand or arm. The contrast dye will be injected through the IV during the scan. You may have a warm feeling when this happens. The dye will highlight your blood vessels on the CT scan pictures.

The technician who runs the cardiac CT scanner will clean areas of your chest and apply sticky patches called electrodes. The patches are attached to an EKG machine to record your heart's electrical activity during the scan.

The CT scanner is a large machine that has a hollow, circular tube in the middle. You will lie on your back on a sliding table. The table can move up and down, and it goes inside the tunnel-like machine.

The table will slowly slide into the opening in the machine. Inside the scanner, an x-ray tube moves around your body to take pictures of different parts of your heart. A computer will put the pictures together to make a 3D picture of the whole heart.

The technician controls the CT scanner from the next room. He or she can see you through a glass window and talk to you through a speaker.

Moving your body can cause the pictures to blur. You'll be asked to lie still and hold your breath for short periods while each picture is taken.

A cardiac CT scan usually takes about 15 minutes to complete. However, it can take more than an hour to get ready for the test and for the medicine to slow your heart rate enough.

What to Expect after Cardiac CT

After the cardiac CT scan, you'll be able to return to your normal activities. A doctor who has experience with CT will provide your doctor with the results of your scan. Your doctor will discuss the findings with you.

Risks of Cardiac CT

Because an x-ray machine is used, cardiac CT involves radiation. Although the amount of radiation used is considered small, it's similar to the amount of radiation you're naturally exposed to over a three-year period.

There's a small chance cardiac CT could cause cancer because of the radiation involved. The risk is higher for people younger than 40 years old, especially children. However, new cardiac CT methods are available that reduce the amount of radiation used for this test.

Cardiac CT scans are painless. Some people feel side effects from the contrast dye sometimes used during the cardiac CT scan. An itchy feeling or rash may appear after the contrast dye is injected. Neither side effect normally lasts for long, so medicine often isn't needed. If you do want medicine to relieve the symptoms, your doctor may prescribe an antihistamine. This type of medicine is used to help stop allergic reactions.

Although rare, it's possible to have a serious allergic reaction to the contrast dye in the form of breathing problems. Medicines are used to treat serious reactions.

People who have asthma, COPD, or heart failure may have breathing problems during cardiac CT if they're given beta blockers to slow down their heart rates.

What Cardiac CT Shows

Cardiac CT is a common test for finding and evaluating the following types of heart problems:

- **Calcium buildup in the walls of the coronary arteries:** This type of CT scan is called a coronary calcium scan. It is discussed in greater detail later in this chapter.

- **CHD:** If contrast dye is used during cardiac CT, it helps highlight the coronary arteries on the x-rays. This can show whether the coronary arteries are narrowed or blocked (which may cause chest pain or a heart attack).

- **Problems with heart function and heart valves:** Doctors may recommend cardiac CT instead of echocardiography or cardiac magnetic resonance imaging for some people.

- **Problems with the aorta:** The aorta is the main artery that carries oxygen-rich blood from the heart to the body. Cardiac CT can detect two serious problems in the aorta: aneurysm and dissection. These problems are discussed in chapter 7, "Aortic Aneurysm."

- **Blood clots in the lungs:** A cardiac CT scan also may be used to find a pulmonary embolism (PE). A PE is a sudden blockage in a lung artery and is usually due to a blood clot that traveled to the lungs from one of the legs. This is a serious but treatable condition.

- **Problems with the pulmonary veins:** The pulmonary veins carry blood from the lungs to the heart. Problems with these veins may lead to atrial fibrillation (AF), an irregular heart rhythm. The pictures that cardiac CT creates of the pulmonary veins can help guide procedures used to treat AF.

- **Pericardial disease:** This is a disease that occurs in the pericardium, the sac around the heart. A cardiac CT takes clear, detailed pictures of the pericardium.

Cardiac CT also may be used before or after certain heart procedures, such as cardiac resynchronization therapy and coronary artery bypass grafting. A cardiac CT can help your doctor pinpoint the areas of the heart or blood vessels where the procedure should be done. The scan also can help your doctor check your heart after the procedure.

Because the heart is in motion, a fast type of CT scanner, called multidetector computed tomography (MDCT), may be used to take high-quality pictures of the heart. MDCT also may be used to detect calcium in the coronary arteries.

Another type of CT scanner, called electron-beam computed tomography (EBCT), also is used to detect calcium in the coronary arteries.

Coronary Calcium Scanning

A coronary calcium scan looks for specks of calcium (called calcifications) in the walls of the coronary arteries. Calcifications are an early sign of CHD. The test can show whether you're at increased risk for a heart attack or other heart problems before other signs and symptoms occur.

Two machines can show calcium in the coronary arteries—EBCT and MDCT. Both use an x-ray machine to make detailed pictures of your heart. Doctors study the pictures to see whether you're at risk for heart problems in the next 2 to 10 years.

A coronary calcium scan is simple and easy for the patient, who lies quietly in the scanner machine for about 10 minutes. The scanner takes pictures of the heart to show whether the coronary arteries have calcifications.

A coronary calcium scan is most useful for people who are at moderate risk for a heart attack. People who are at moderate risk have a 10 to 20% chance of having a heart attack within the next 10 years. The coronary calcium scan may help doctors decide who within this group needs treatment.

What to Expect before a Coronary Calcium Scan

No special preparation is needed for a coronary calcium scan. Your doctor may ask you to avoid caffeine and smoking for four hours before the test.

For the scan, you'll remove your clothes above the waist and wear a hospital gown. You also will remove any jewelry from around your neck or chest.

What to Expect during a Coronary Calcium Scan

Coronary calcium scans are done in a hospital or outpatient office. The x-ray machine that's used is called a CT scanner, and the test is done in the same way as a cardiac CT scan.

As with a cardiac CT scan, you'll be asked to lie still and hold your breath for short periods while each picture is taken. You may be given medicine to slow down a fast heart rate, which helps the machine take better pictures of your heart. The medicine will be given by mouth or injected into a vein.

A coronary calcium scan takes about 10 to 15 minutes, although the actual scanning takes only a few seconds. During the test, the machine makes clicking and whirring sounds as it takes pictures. It causes no discomfort, but the exam room may be chilly to keep the machine working properly.

If you become nervous in enclosed spaces, you may need to take medicine to stay calm. This isn't a problem for most people because the patient's head remains outside the opening in the machine.

What to Expect after a Coronary Calcium Scan

You'll be able to return to your normal activities after the coronary calcium scan is done. Your doctor will discuss the results of the calcium scan with you.

Risks of Coronary Calcium Scanning

Coronary calcium scanning has very few risks. The test isn't invasive, which means no surgery is done and no instruments are inserted into your body.

Coronary calcium scanning doesn't require an injection of contrast dye to make your heart or arteries visible on x-ray images.

Because an x-ray machine is used, you'll be exposed to a small amount of radiation. EBCT uses less radiation than MDCT. In either case, the amount of radiation is less than or equal to the amount of radiation you're naturally exposed to in a single year.

What a Coronary Calcium Scan Shows

After a coronary calcium scan, you'll get a calcium score called an Agatston score. The score is based on the amount of calcium found in your coronary (heart) arteries. You may get an Agatston score for each major artery and a total score.

The test is negative if no calcium deposits (calcifications) are found in your arteries. This means your chance of having a heart attack in the next two to five years is low.

The test is positive if calcifications are found in your arteries. Calcifications are a sign of atherosclerosis and CHD. (Atherosclerosis is a condition in which the arteries harden and narrow due to plaque buildup.) The higher your Agatston score, the more severe your atherosclerosis.

An Agatston score of 0 is normal. In general, the higher your score, the more likely you are to have CHD. If your score is high, your doctor may recommend more tests.

Cardiac Magnetic Resonance Imaging

Magnetic resonance imaging (MRI) is a safe, noninvasive test that creates detailed pictures of your organs and tissues. Noninvasive means no surgery is done and no instruments are inserted into your body.

MRI uses radio waves, magnets, and a computer to create pictures of your organs and tissues. Unlike CT scans and standard x-rays, MRI doesn't use ionizing radiation or carry any risk of causing cancer.

Cardiac MRI creates pictures of your heart as it's beating, producing both still and moving pictures of your heart and major blood vessels. Doctors use cardiac MRI to get pictures of the beating heart and to look at its structure and function. These pictures can help them decide how to treat people who have heart problems.

Cardiac MRI can help explain results from other tests, such as x-rays and CT scans. Sometimes, cardiac MRI is used to avoid invasive procedures or tests that use radiation (such as x-rays) or dyes containing iodine (these dyes may be harmful to people who have kidney problems).

Often during cardiac MRI, a contrast agent is injected into a vein to highlight portions of the heart or blood vessels. This contrast agent often is used for people who are allergic to the dyes used in CT scanning.

People who have severe kidney or liver problems may not be able to have the contrast agent. As a result, they may have an MRI that doesn't use the substance (a noncontrast MRI).

What to Expect before Cardiac MRI

You'll be asked to fill out a screening form before having cardiac MRI. The form may ask whether you have had previous surgeries, have any metal objects in your body, or have any medical devices (like a cardiac pacemaker) surgically implanted in your body.

Most, but not all, implanted medical devices are allowed near MRI machines. Talk to your doctor or the technician operating the machine if you have concerns about any implanted devices or conditions that may interfere with the MRI.

MRI can seriously affect some types of implanted medical devices:

- Implanted cardiac pacemakers and defibrillators can malfunction.

- Cochlear (inner-ear) implants can be damaged. Cochlear implants are small electronic devices that help people who are deaf or who can't hear well understand speech and the sounds around them.

- Brain aneurysm clips can move due to the MRI machine's strong magnetic field. This can cause severe injury.

Your doctor will let you know if you shouldn't have a cardiac MRI because of a medical device. If this applies to you, consider wearing a medical identification bracelet or necklace or carrying a medical alert card stating you shouldn't have an MRI.

Your doctor or technician will tell you whether you need to change into a hospital gown for the test. Don't bring hearing aids, credit cards, jewelry or watches, eyeglasses, pens, removable dental work, or anything that's magnetic near the MRI machine.

Tell your doctor if being in a fairly tight or confined space causes you anxiety or fear. This fear is called claustrophobia. If you have this condition, your doctor might give you medicine to help you relax. Your doctor may ask you to fast (not eat) for six hours before you take this medicine on the day of the test.

Some of the newer cardiac MRI machines are open on all sides. Ask your doctor to help you find a facility that has an open MRI machine if you're fearful in tight or confined spaces.

Your doctor will let you know whether you need to arrange for a ride home after the test.

What to Expect during Cardiac MRI

MRI machines usually are located in hospitals or special medical imaging facilities. A radiologist or other doctor who has special training in medical imaging oversees MRI testing.

Cardiac MRI usually takes 45 to 90 minutes, depending on how many pictures are needed. The test may take less time with some newer MRI machines.

MRI machines are located in specially constructed rooms that prevent radio waves from disrupting the machine. These rooms also prevent the MRI machine's strong magnetic fields from interfering with other equipment.

Traditional MRI machines look like long, narrow tunnels. Newer MRI machines, called short-bore systems, are shorter, wider, and don't completely surround you. Some of the newer machines are open on all sides. Your doctor will help decide which type of machine is best for you.

Cardiac MRI is painless and harmless. You'll lie on your back on a sliding table that goes inside the tunnel-like machine. The technician will control the machine from the next room. He or she will be able to see you through a glass window and talk to you through a speaker. Tell the technician if you have a hearing problem.

The MRI machine makes loud humming, tapping, and buzzing noises. Earplugs may help lessen the noises made by the MRI machine. Some facilities let you listen to music during the test.

You will need to remain very still during the test. Any movement may blur the pictures. If you're unable to lie still, you may be given medicine to help you relax.

You may be asked to hold your breath for 10 to 15 seconds at a time while the technician takes pictures of your heart. Researchers are studying ways to allow someone having a cardiac MRI to breathe freely during the exam while achieving the same image quality.

A contrast agent, such as gadolinium, may be used to highlight your blood vessels or heart in the pictures. The contrast agent usually is injected into a vein in your arm with a needle.

You may feel a cool sensation during the injection and discomfort where the needle was inserted. Gadolinium doesn't contain iodine, so it won't cause problems for people who are allergic to iodine.

Your cardiac MRI may include a stress test to detect blockages in your coronary arteries. If so, you'll get other medicines to increase the blood flow in your heart or increase your heart rate.

What to Expect after Cardiac MRI

If you weren't given medicine to help you relax, you'll be able to return to your normal routine after the cardiac MRI. If you did take medicine to help you relax during the test, your doctor will tell you when you can return to your normal routine. You'll need someone to drive you home.

Risks of Cardiac MRI

Cardiac MRI produces no side effects from the magnetic fields and radio waves. This method of taking pictures of organs and tissues doesn't carry a risk of causing cancer or birth defects.

Serious reactions to the contrast agent used for MRI are very rare. However, side effects are possible and include headache, nausea, dizziness, changes in taste, and allergic reactions. Rarely, the contrast agent can be harmful in people who have severe kidney or liver disease. It may cause a disease called nephrogenic systemic fibrosis.

If your cardiac MRI includes a stress test, more medicines will be used during the test. These medicines may have other side effects that aren't expected during a regular MRI scan, such as arrhythmias (irregular heartbeats), chest pain, shortness of breath, or palpitations (feeling your heart is skipping a beat, fluttering, or beating too hard or fast).

What Cardiac MRI Shows

The doctor supervising your scan will provide your doctor with the results of your cardiac MRI. Your doctor will discuss the findings with you.

Cardiac MRI can reveal a number of heart conditions and disorders, including coronary heart disease, damage caused by a heart attack, heart failure, heart valve problems, congenital heart defects, pericarditis (a condition in which the membrane, or sac, around your heart is inflamed), and cardiac tumors.

Cardiac MRI is a fast, accurate tool that can help diagnose a heart attack by detecting areas of the heart that don't move normally, have poor blood supply, or are scarred.

Cardiac MRI can show whether any of the coronary arteries are blocked, causing reduced blood flow to your heart muscle. Coronary angiography, described in chapter 14, is an invasive procedure that uses x-rays and iodine-based dyes. Researchers have found that cardiac MRI can replace coronary angiography in some cases, avoiding the need to use x-ray radiation and iodine-based dyes. This use of MRI is called MRI angiography.

Researchers are finding new ways to use cardiac MRI. In the future, cardiac MRI may replace x-rays as the main way to guide invasive procedures such as cardiac catheterization. Also, improvements in cardiac MRI are likely to lead to better methods for detecting heart disease in the future.

Adapted from "Cardiac CT" and "Coronary Calcium Scan," November 2009, with additional information excerpted from "Cardiac MRI," July 2009, all three produced by the National Heart, Lung, and Blood Institute (NHLBI, www.nhlbi .nih.gov).

Chapter 14

Coronary Angiograms and Cardiac Catheterization

Coronary Angiography

Coronary angiography is a test that uses dye and special x-rays to show the inside of your coronary arteries, the arteries that supply oxygen-rich blood to your heart. Coronary angiography is the most accurate method to determine whether you have coronary heart disease (CHD), but it is also the most invasive.

Most of the time, the coronary arteries can't be seen on an x-ray. During coronary angiography, a special dye is injected into the bloodstream to make the coronary arteries show up on an x-ray. A procedure called cardiac catheterization is used to get the dye to your coronary arteries.

Cardiac Catheterization

Cardiac catheterization is a medical procedure used to diagnose and treat certain heart conditions. A long, thin, flexible tube called a catheter is put into a blood vessel in your arm, groin (upper thigh), or neck and threaded to your heart. Through the catheter, doctors can do diagnostic tests and treatments on your heart.

For example, in coronary angiography your doctor will put a special dye in the catheter. This dye will flow through your bloodstream to your heart. Once the dye reaches your heart, it will make the inside of your coronary (heart) arteries show up on an x-ray. The dye can show whether plaque has narrowed or blocked any of your coronary arteries.

Blockages in the coronary arteries also can be seen using ultrasound during cardiac catheterization. Ultrasound uses sound waves to create detailed pictures of the heart's blood vessels.

Doctors may take samples of blood and heart muscle during cardiac catheterization and do minor heart surgery.

Cardiologists (heart specialists) usually do cardiac catheterization in a hospital. You're awake during the procedure, and it causes little to no pain. However, you may feel some soreness in the blood vessel where the catheter was inserted. Cardiac catheterization rarely causes serious complications.

When Coronary Angiography or Cardiac Catheterization Is Necessary

Coronary Angiography

Your doctor may recommend coronary angiography if you have signs or symptoms of CHD, such as angina or sudden cardiac arrest. Coronary angiography may also be recommended if results from an EKG, exercise stress test, or other test suggest you have heart disease.

You also may need coronary angiography on an emergency basis if you're having a heart attack. This test, combined with a procedure called angioplasty, can open the blocked artery causing the heart attack and prevent further damage to your heart.

Coronary angiography also can help your doctor decide how to treat CHD after a heart attack. This is especially true if the heart attack caused major damage to your heart or if you're still having chest pain.

Cardiac Catheterization

Cardiac catheterization is used to diagnose and treat many heart conditions. Doctors may recommend this procedure for various reasons. The most common reason is to evaluate chest pain. Chest pain may be a symptom of CHD. Cardiac catheterization can show whether plaque is narrowing or blocking your heart's arteries.

Doctors can treat CHD during cardiac catheterization with a procedure called angioplasty. During angioplasty, a tiny balloon is put through the catheter and into the blocked artery. When the balloon is inflated, it pushes the plaque against the artery wall, which creates a wider pathway for blood to flow to the heart. Angioplasty is discussed in chapter 22.

Most people who suffer heart attacks have partly or completely blocked coronary arteries. Thus, cardiac catheterization may be done on an emergency basis while you're having a heart attack. When used with angioplasty, the procedure allows your doctor to open blocked arteries and prevent more damage to your heart.

Cardiac catheterization also can help your doctor figure out the best treatment for your CHD if you have recently recovered from a heart attack but are having chest pain. It can also help if you have had a heart attack that caused major damage to your heart or if you have had an EKG, stress test, or other test that suggested heart disease.

You also may need cardiac catheterization if your doctor suspects you have a heart defect or if you're about to have heart surgery. The procedure shows the overall shape of your heart and the four large spaces (heart chambers) inside it. This inside view of the heart will show certain heart defects and help your doctor plan your heart surgery.

Sometimes doctors do cardiac catheterization to see how well the valves at the openings and exits of the heart chambers are working. Valves control the flow of blood in the heart.

To check your valves, your doctor will measure blood flow and oxygen levels in different parts of your heart. Cardiac catheterization also can check how well a man-made heart valve is working and how well your heart is pumping blood.

If your doctor thinks you have a heart infection or tumor, he or she may take samples of your heart muscle through the catheter. With the help of cardiac catheterization, doctors can even do minor heart surgery, such as repairing certain heart defects.

What to Expect before Coronary Angiography or Cardiac Catheterization

Before having coronary angiography or cardiac catheterization, talk to your doctor about how the test is done and how to prepare for it. Discuss any medicines you're taking and whether you should stop taking them before the test. If you have diabetes, kidney disease, or other conditions, you may need to take extra steps during or after the test to avoid complications

Your doctor will tell you exactly which procedures will be done. You will have the chance to ask questions about the procedure. Also, you'll be asked to provide written informed consent to have the procedures done.

It may not be safe to drive after having cardiac catheterization, which is also a part of coronary angiography, so you must arrange for a ride home.

What to Expect during Coronary Angiography or Cardiac Catheterization

Coronary angiography and cardiac catheterization are done in a hospital. During the procedure you'll be kept on your back and awake so you can follow your doctor's instructions during the test. You'll be given medicine to help you relax. The medicine may make you sleepy.

Your doctor will numb the area on your arm, groin (upper thigh), or neck where the catheter will enter your blood vessel. A needle is used to make a small hole in the blood vessel. Your doctor will put a tapered tube called a sheath through this hole.

Next, your doctor will put a thin, flexible wire through the sheath and into your blood vessel. This guide wire is then threaded through your blood vessel to your heart. The wire helps your doctor position the catheter correctly. Your doctor then puts a catheter through the sheath and slides it over the guide wire and into the coronary arteries.

Special x-ray movies will be taken of the catheter as it's moved up into the heart. The movies will help your doctor see where to position the tip of the catheter.

During coronary angiography, your doctor will put a special dye in the catheter to make the inside of your heart's arteries show up on an x-ray. Coronary angiography can show how well blood is being pumped out of the heart's main pumping chambers, called ventricles.

While the catheter is inside your heart, your doctor may use it to take blood samples from different parts of the heart or do minor heart surgery.

To get a more detailed view of a blocked coronary artery, your doctor may do an intracoronary ultrasound. For this test, your doctor will thread a tiny ultrasound device through the catheter and into the artery. This device gives off sound waves that bounce off the artery wall (and its blockage) to make an image of the inside of the artery.

If the angiogram or intracoronary ultrasound shows blockages or other possible problems in the heart's arteries, your doctor may use angioplasty to open the blocked arteries.

After your doctor does all the needed tests or treatments, he or she will pull back the catheter and take it out along with the sheath. The opening in the blood vessel will then be closed up and bandaged. A small weight may be put on top of the bandage for a few hours to apply more pressure. This will help prevent major bleeding from the site.

What to Expect after Coronary Angiography or Cardiac Catheterization

After coronary angiography or cardiac catheterization, you'll be moved to a special care area, where you'll rest and be checked for several hours or overnight. During this time, you'll need to limit your movement to avoid bleeding from the site where the catheter was inserted.

While you recover in the special care area, nurses will check your heart rate and blood pressure regularly and note whether you're bleeding from the tube insertion site.

A bruise may develop on your arm, groin, or neck at the site where the catheter was inserted. In some cases, the bruise may be quite large and may slowly spread downward over several days. That area may feel sore or tender for about a week. Let your doctor know if you develop constant or heavy bleeding at the catheter insertion site that can't be stopped with a small bandage or any unusual pain, swelling, redness, or other signs of infection at or near the catheter insertion site.

Talk to your doctor about whether you should avoid certain activities, such as heavy lifting, for a short time after the test.

Risks of Coronary Angiography and Cardiac Catheterization

Coronary angiography and cardiac catheterization are common medical tests that rarely cause serious problems, but complications sometimes occur. They can include bleeding, infection, and pain at the site where the catheter was inserted or damage to blood vessels. Also, in some people an allergic reaction to the dye can occur.

Other less common complications of the test include the following:

- An arrhythmia (irregular heartbeat) that often goes away on its own but may need treatment if it persists

- Damage to the kidneys caused by the dye used

- Blood clots that can trigger stroke, heart attack, or other serious problems

- Low blood pressure

- A buildup of blood or fluid in the sac that surrounds the heart (this fluid can prevent the heart from beating properly)

As with any procedure involving the heart, complications can sometimes be fatal. However, this is rare with coronary angiography or cardiac catheterization.

The risk of complications from coronary angiography or cardiac catheterization is higher if you have diabetes or kidney disease or if you're 75 years old or older. The risk of complications also is greater in women and in people having the procedure on an emergency basis.

Excerpted and adapted from "Coronary Angiography" and "Cardiac Catheterization," May 2009, both produced by the National Heart, Lung, and Blood Institute (NHLBI, www.nhlbi.nih.gov).

Chapter 15

Catheter Ablation

Catheter ablation is a medical procedure used to treat some types of arrhythmia. Arrhythmias are explained in chapter 4. During catheter ablation, a special tube is guided into your heart through a blood vessel. A machine sends energy through the ablation catheter to your heart. The energy destroys small areas of heart tissue where abnormal heartbeats may cause an arrhythmia to start.

Radiofrequency (RF) energy usually is used for catheter ablation. This type of energy uses radio waves to produce heat that destroys the heart tissue. Studies have shown that RF energy is safe and effective.

Cardiologists (heart specialists) sometimes do ablation during open-heart surgery. This method isn't as common as catheter ablation, which doesn't require surgery to open the chest.

Catheter ablation alone doesn't always restore a normal heart rate and rhythm. You may need other treatments as well. Also, some people who have the procedure may need to have it done again. This can happen if the first procedure doesn't fully correct the problem.

Other Names for Catheter Ablation

- Ablation
- Cardiac ablation
- Cardiac catheter ablation
- Radiofrequency ablation
- Catheter cryoablation

When Catheter Ablation Is Necessary

Your doctor may recommend catheter ablation for certain types of arrhythmia, if you have an arrhythmia medicine can't control, or if you can't tolerate the medicines your doctor has prescribed for your arrhythmia. If you have abnormal electrical activity in your heart that raises your risk of a life-threatening arrhythmia, your doctor may also recommend catheter ablation.

What to Expect before Catheter Ablation

Before you have catheter ablation, your doctor may review your medical history, do a physical exam, and recommend tests and procedures.

Your doctor will want to know about any medicines you're taking. Some medicines can interfere with catheter ablation. If you take any of these medicines, your doctor may advise you to stop taking them before the procedure.

Your doctor also may ask whether you have diabetes, kidney disease, or other conditions. If so, your doctor may need to take extra steps during or after the procedure to help you avoid complications.

If you're pregnant, let your doctor know before having catheter ablation. The procedure involves radiation, which can harm a fetus. Talk with your doctor about whether you should have the procedure or wait. If you're a woman of childbearing age, your doctor may recommend a pregnancy test before catheter ablation to make sure you're not pregnant.

Once the procedure is scheduled, your doctor will tell you how to prepare for it. You'll likely need to stop eating and drinking by midnight before the procedure. Your doctor will give you specific instructions.

Some people go home the day of the procedure. Others need to stay overnight for one or more days. Driving after the procedure may not be safe. Your doctor will let you know whether you need to arrange for someone to drive you home.

What to Expect during Catheter Ablation

Catheter ablation is done in a hospital. Doctors who do this procedure have special training in cardiac electrophysiology (the heart's electrical system) and ablation (destruction) of diseased heart tissue.

Before the Procedure

Before the procedure, you'll be given medicine through an IV line inserted into a vein in your arm. The medicine will help you relax. It may make you sleepy. You'll also be connected to several machines that will check your heart's activity during the procedure.

Once you're drowsy, your doctor will numb an area on your arm, groin, or neck. A needle will be used to make a small hole through your skin and into a blood vessel. Your doctor will put a tapered tube called a sheath through this hole.

Your doctor will then put a thin, flexible guide wire and an ablation catheter (a long, thin, flexible tube) through the sheath and into your blood vessel. The guide wire will be threaded through your blood vessel and into your heart. The wire will help your doctor place the catheter correctly.

Your doctor will then put a special dye into the catheter. The dye will make the inside of your heart show up on special x-ray images called angiograms. The images will help your doctor place the tip of the catheter at the correct spot in your heart.

During the Procedure

Electrodes at the end of the catheter will be used to stimulate your heart and record its electrical activity. This will help your doctor learn where abnormal heartbeats are starting in your heart.

Your doctor will aim the tip of the catheter at the small area of heart tissue where the abnormal heartbeats are starting. A special machine will send energy through the catheter to create a scar line, also called an ablation line.

The scar line will create a barrier between the damaged heart tissue and the surrounding healthy heart tissue. This will stop abnormal electrical signals from traveling to the rest of the heart and causing arrhythmias.

What You May Feel

You may sleep on and off during the procedure. You generally will not feel anything except a burning sensation when your doctor injects medicine into the area where the catheter will be inserted, discomfort or burning in your chest when the energy is applied, or a faster heartbeat during studies that pinpoint the area(s) of your heart where abnormal heartbeats are starting.

The procedure lasts three to six hours. When the procedure is done, your doctor will pull back and remove the ablation catheter along with the sheath and guide wire.

The opening in the blood vessel will be closed and bandaged. Nurses will apply pressure to this site to help prevent major bleeding and help the area begin to heal.

What to Expect after Catheter Ablation

After catheter ablation, you'll be moved to a special care unit where you'll lie still for four to six hours of recovery. Lying still prevents bleeding at the site where the ablation catheter was inserted.

While you're in the special care unit, you'll be connected to special devices that measure your heart's electrical activity and blood pressure. Nurses will check these monitors regularly. Nurses also will check to make sure you're not bleeding from the catheter insertion site.

Going Home

Your doctor will decide whether you need to stay overnight in the hospital. Some people go home the day of the procedure. Others need to stay in the hospital for one or more days.

Before you go home, your doctor will tell you which medicines you need to take, how much physical activity you can do, how to care for the area where the catheter was inserted, and when to schedule follow-up care.

Driving after the procedure may not be safe. Your doctor will let you know whether you need to arrange for someone to drive you home.

Recovery and Recuperation

Recovery from catheter ablation usually is quick. You may feel stiff and achy from lying still for four to six hours after the procedure. Also, a small bruise may form at the site where the catheter was inserted. The area may feel sore or tender for about a week. Most people are able to return to normal activities in a few days.

Your doctor will talk with you about signs and symptoms to watch for. Let your doctor know if you have any of the following problems:

- Constant or heavy bleeding at the catheter insertion site that you can't stop with a small bandage

- Unusual pain, swelling, redness, or other signs of infection at or near the catheter insertion site

- Strong, rapid, or other irregular heartbeats

- Fainting

Risks of Catheter Ablation

Catheter ablation has some risks. The procedure may cause any of the following:

- Bleeding, infection, and pain at the site where the ablation catheter was inserted

- Damage to your blood vessels; although this complication is very rare, it's caused by the catheter scraping or poking a hole in a blood vessel as it's guided to the heart

- Puncture of the heart

- Damage to the heart's electrical system, which may cause you to need a permanent pacemaker (a small device that's placed under the skin of your chest or abdomen to help control abnormal heart rhythms)

- Blood clots, which could lead to stroke or other complications

- Narrowing of the veins that carry blood from the lungs to the heart, called stenosis

As with any heart procedure, complications can sometimes be fatal. However, this is rare with catheter ablation. The risk of complications is higher if you have diabetes or kidney disease. The risk also is higher if you're 75 years old or older.

Adapted from "Catheter Ablation," National Heart, Lung, and Blood Institute (NHLBI, www.nhlbi.nih.gov), February 2010.

Chapter 16

An Aspirin a Day?

You can walk into any pharmacy, grocery, or convenience store and buy aspirin without a prescription. The Drug Facts label on medication products will help you choose aspirin for relieving headache, pain, swelling, or fever. The Drug Facts label also gives directions to help you use the aspirin so that it is safe and effective.

But what about using aspirin for a different use, for a different time period, or in a manner not listed on the label? For example, using aspirin to lower the risk of heart attack and clot-related strokes. In these cases, the labeling information does not help you choose or use the medicine safely. Since you don't have labeling directions to help you, you need the medical knowledge of your doctor, nurse practitioner, or other health professional.

You can increase the chance of getting the good effects and decrease the chance of getting the bad effects of any medicine by choosing and using it wisely. When it comes to using aspirin to lower the risk of heart attack and stroke, choosing and using wisely means knowing the facts and working with your health professional.

Daily Use of Aspirin Is Not Right for Everyone

Aspirin has been shown to be helpful when used daily to lower the risk of heart attack, clot-related strokes, and other blood-flow problems. Many medical professionals prescribe aspirin for these uses. There may be a benefit to daily aspirin use if you have some kind of heart or blood vessel disease or if you have evidence of poor blood flow to the brain. However, the risks of long-term aspirin use may be greater than the benefits if there are no signs of or risk factors for heart or blood vessel disease.

Every prescription and over-the-counter medicine has benefits and risks—even common and familiar medicines such as aspirin. Aspirin use can result in serious side effects, such as stomach bleeding, bleeding in the brain, kidney failure, and some kinds of strokes. No medicine is completely safe. By carefully reviewing many different factors, your health professional can help you make the best choice for you.

When you don't have labeling directions to guide you, you need the medical knowledge of your doctor, nurse practitioner, or other health professional.

Aspirin Is a Drug

If you are at risk for heart attack or stroke your doctor may prescribe aspirin to increase blood flow to your heart and brain. But any drug—including aspirin—can have harmful side effects, especially when mixed with other products. In fact, the chance of side effects increases with each new product you use.

New products include prescription and other over-the-counter medicines, dietary supplement (including vitamins and herbals), and sometimes foods and beverages. For instance, people who already use a prescribed blood thinner should not use aspirin unless recommended by a health professional. There are also dietary supplements known to thin the blood. Using aspirin with alcohol or with another product that also contains aspirin, such as a cough-sinus drug, can increase the chance of side effects.

Your health professional will consider your current state of health. Some medical conditions, such as pregnancy, uncontrolled high blood pressure, bleeding disorders, asthma, peptic (stomach) ulcers, and liver and kidney disease, could make aspirin a bad choice for you.

Make sure all your health professionals are aware you are using aspirin to reduce your risk of heart attack and clot-related strokes.

Safe Use of Aspirin Depends on Following Your Doctor's Directions

There are no directions on the label for using aspirin to reduce the risk of heart attack or clot-related stroke. You may rely on your health professional to provide the correct information on dose and directions for use. Using aspirin correctly gives you the best chance of getting the greatest benefits with the fewest unwanted side effects. Discuss with your health professional the different forms of aspirin products that might be best suited for you.

Aspirin has been shown to lower the risk of heart attack and stroke, but not all over-the-counter pain and fever reducers have this effect. Even though the directions on the aspirin label do not apply to this use of aspirin, you still need to read the label to confirm the product you buy and use contains aspirin at the correct dose. Check the Drug Facts label for "active ingredients: aspirin" or "acetylsalicylic acid" at the dose your health professional has prescribed.

Remember, if you are using aspirin every day for weeks, months, or years to prevent a heart attack or stroke or for any use not listed on the label without the guidance of your health professional, you could be doing your body more harm than good.

The Value and Risks of Taking Aspirin Differ for Men and Women

The U.S. Preventive Services Task Force recently issued separate recommendations for men and women on taking aspirin to prevent cardiovascular disease. The task force is a leading independent panel of experts in prevention and primary care.

The new task force recommendations are based on recent research indicating the value of taking aspirin differs for men and women. For men, the benefit of taking aspirin is that it lowers the risk of heart attack. For women, it lowers the risk of stroke.

The task force also looked at recent evidence on the potential harmful effects of taking aspirin, like bleeding in the stomach. These risks vary for men and women, for different ages, and depending on other factors, such as the use of other medications.

Taking into account the potential benefits and harms, the task force recommends the following:

- If you're a man who is 45 to 79 years old, you should talk to your doctor to determine whether the benefits of taking aspirin to prevent a heart attack outweigh the potential harms.

- If you're a woman who 55 to 79 years old, you should talk to your doctor to determine whether the benefits of taking aspirin to prevent a stroke outweigh the potential harms.

Why are these recommendations important? Because they help you and your clinician make informed decisions about what you can do to stay healthy.

It's important for men and women to ask questions about their risks for heart attack and stroke. Understanding your risk for cardiovascular disease can help you take steps to reduce your risk and possibly prevent heart problems or stroke.

Getting advice specific to you will help you become a better-informed patient. And that's good news for your health over the long run, whether you're a man or a woman.

Adapted from "Aspirin for Reducing Your Risk of Heart Attack and Stroke: Know the Facts," U.S. Food and Drug Administration (FDA, www.fda.gov), April 30, 2009, and "An Aspirin a Day? The Answer Is Different for Men and Women," Agency for Healthcare Research and Quality (AHRQ, www.ahrq.gov), August 4, 2009.

Chapter 17

Using Blood Thinners Safely

About Your Blood Thinner

Your doctor may prescribe a medicine called a blood thinner to prevent blood clots. Blood clots can put you at risk for heart attack, stroke, and other serious medical problems. A blood thinner is a kind of drug called an anticoagulant. *Anti* means against and *coagulant* means to thicken into a gel or solid.

How to Take Your Blood Thinner

Always take your blood thinner as directed. For example, some blood thinners need to be taken at the same time of day, every day.

Never skip a dose, and never take a double dose.

If you miss a dose, take it as soon as you remember. If you don't remember until the next day, call your doctor for instructions. If this happens when your doctor is not available, skip the missed dose and start again the next day. Mark the missed dose in a diary or on a calendar.

A pillbox with a slot for each day may help you keep track of your medicines.

> **Warning!**
>
> Tell your doctor if you are pregnant or plan to get pregnant. Many blood thinners can cause birth defects or bleeding that may harm your unborn child.

Check Your Medicine

Check your medicine when you get it from the pharmacy:

- Does the medicine seem different from what your doctor prescribed or look different from what you expected?

- Does your pill look different from what you used before?

- Are the color, shape, and markings on the pill the same as what you were previously given?

If something seems different, ask the pharmacist to double-check it. Many medication errors are found by patients.

Using Other Medicines

Tell your doctor about every medicine you take. The doctor needs to know about all your medicines, including medicines you were taking before you started taking a blood thinner.

Other medicines can change the way your blood thinner works. Your blood thinner can also change the way your other medicines work.

Most antibiotics will affect how your blood thinner works. You should always make sure the person prescribing your antibiotic is aware you are taking a blood thinner. You may need to have your blood thinner dose adjusted or have more frequent blood testing performed.

It is very important to talk with your doctor about all the medicines you take, including other prescription medicines, over-the-counter medicines, vitamins, and herbal products.

Products that contain aspirin may lessen the blood's ability to form clots and may increase your risk of bleeding when you also are taking a blood thinner. Talk with your doctor about whether or not you should take aspirin and which dose is right for you.

Medicines you get over-the-counter may also interact with your blood thinner. Talk with your doctor before using any of the following common pain relievers, cold medicines, or stomach remedies:

- Advil®
- Aleve®
- Alka-Seltzer®
- Excedrin®
- Ex-lax®
- Midol®
- Motrin®
- Nuprin®
- Pamprin HB®
- Pepto-Bismol®
- Sine-Off®
- Tagamet HB®
- Tylenol®

Also talk with your doctor before using any of the following vitamins and herbal products:

- Centrum®, One a Day®, or other multivitamins
- Garlic
- Ginkgo biloba
- Green tea
- St. John's wort

Always tell your doctor about all the medicines you are taking. Tell your doctor when you start taking new medicine, when you stop taking a medicine, or if the amount of medicine you are taking changes. When you visit your doctor, bring a list of current medicines, over-the-counter drugs such as aspirin, and any vitamins or herbal products you take.

Possible Side Effects

When taking a blood thinner it is important to be aware of its possible side effects. Bleeding is the most common side effect.

Call your doctor immediately if you have any of the following signs of serious bleeding:

- Menstrual bleeding that is much heavier than normal
- Red or brown urine
- Bowel movements that are red or look like tar
- Bleeding from the gums or nose that does not stop quickly
- Vomit that is brown or bright red
- Anything red in color that you cough up
- Severe pain, such as a headache or stomachache
- Unusual bruising
- A cut that does not stop bleeding
- A serious fall or bump on the head
- Dizziness or weakness

Some people who take a blood thinner may experience hair loss or skin rashes, but this is rare.

Stay Safe While Taking Your Blood Thinner

Call your doctor and go to the hospital immediately if you have a bad fall or a hard bump, even if you are not bleeding. You can be bleeding even if you don't see any blood. For example, if you fall and hit your head, bleeding can occur inside your skull. Or if you hurt your arm during a fall and then notice a large purple bruise, you are bleeding under your skin.

Because you are taking a blood thinner, you should try not to hurt yourself and cause bleeding. You need to be careful when you use knives, scissors, razors, or any sharp objects that can make you bleed.

You also need to avoid activities and sports that could cause injury. Swimming and walking are safe activities. If you would like to start a new activity that will increase the amount of exercise you get every day, talk to your doctor.

You can still do many things you enjoy. If you like to work in the yard, you still can. Just be sure to wear sturdy shoes and gloves to protect yourself. Or if you like to bike, be sure to wear a helmet.

Tell others you are using a blood thinner. Keep a current list of all the medicines you take. Ask your doctor about whether you should wear a medical alert bracelet or necklace. If you are badly injured and unable to speak, the bracelet lets health care workers know you are taking a blood thinner.

To prevent injury indoors, use the following precautions:

- Be very careful using knives and scissors.
- Use an electric razor.
- Use a soft toothbrush.
- Use waxed dental floss.
- Do not use toothpicks.
- Wear shoes or nonskid slippers in the house.
- Be careful when you trim your toenails.
- Do not trim corns or calluses yourself.

To prevent injury outdoors, use the following precautions:

- Always wear shoes.
- Wear gloves when using sharp tools.
- Avoid activities and sports that can easily hurt you.
- Wear gardening gloves when doing yard work.

Food and Your Blood Thinner

The foods you eat can affect how well your blood thinner works for you. High amounts of vitamin K might work against some blood thinners, like warfarin (Coumadin®). Other blood thinners are not affected by vitamin K. Ask your doctor if you need to pay attention to the amount of vitamin K you eat.

Examples of foods that contain medium to high levels of vitamin K and can affect your blood thinner are as follows:

- Asparagus
- Avocado
- Broccoli
- Brussels sprouts
- Cabbage
- Canola oil
- Cranberries
- Endive
- Green onions
- Kale
- Lettuce
- Liver
- Margarine
- Mayonnaise
- Parsley
- Soybean oil
- Soybeans
- Spinach
- Turnip, collard, and mustard greens

Call your doctor if you are unable to eat for several days, for whatever reason. Also call if you have stomach problems, vomiting, or diarrhea that lasts more than one day. These problems could affect your blood thinner dose.

Do not make any major changes in your diet or start a weight-loss plan before calling your doctor first.

If you are taking a blood thinner, you should avoid drinking alcohol.

Talk to Your Other Doctors

Because you take a blood thinner, you will be seen regularly by the doctor who prescribed the medicine. You may also see other doctors for different problems. When you see other doctors, it is very important to tell them you are taking a blood thinner. You should also tell your dentist and the person who cleans your teeth.

If you use different pharmacies, make sure each pharmacist knows you take a blood thinner.

Blood thinners can interact with medicines and treatments other doctors might prescribe for you. If another doctor orders a new medicine for you, tell the doctor who ordered your blood thinner because dose changes for your blood thinner may be needed.

Blood Tests

You might have to have your blood tested often if you are taking a blood thinner. The blood test helps your doctor decide how much medicine you need.

The international normalized ratio (INR) blood test measures how fast your blood clots and lets the doctor know if your dose needs to be changed. Testing your blood helps your doctor keep you in a safe range. If there is too much blood thinner in your body, you could bleed too much. If there is not enough, you could get a blood clot.

Once the blood test is in the target range and the correct dose is reached, this test is done less often. Because your dose is based on the INR blood test, it is very important you get your blood tested on the date and at the time you are told.

Illness can affect your INR blood test and your blood thinner dose. If you become sick with a fever, the flu, or an infection, call your doctor. Also call if you have diarrhea or vomiting lasting more than one day.

Adapted from "Blood Thinner Pills: Using Them Safely," Agency for Healthcare Research and Quality (AHRQ, www.ahrq.gov), September 2009.

Chapter 18

Medicines to Manage Blood Pressure

Today's blood pressure medicines can safely help most people control their blood pressure. These medicines are easy to take. The side effects, if any, tend to be minor.

If you have side effects from your medicines, talk to your doctor. He or she may be able to adjust the dose or prescribe other medicines. You shouldn't decide on your own to stop taking your medicine.

Blood pressure medicines work in different ways to lower blood pressure. Some remove extra fluid and salt from the body to lower blood pressure. Others slow down the heartbeat or relax and widen blood vessels. Often, two or more medicines work better than one.

Types of Blood Pressure Medications

There are a number of different medications used to manage blood pressure:

- **Diuretics:** Diuretics are sometimes called water pills. They help your kidneys flush excess water and salt from your body, which lessens the amount of fluid in your blood, causing your blood pressure to go down. Diuretics often are used with other blood pressure medicines and are sometimes combined into one pill.

- **Beta blockers:** Beta blockers help your heart beat slower and with less force and also relax blood vessel walls. This makes your blood pressure goes down.

- **Angiotensin-converting enzyme (ACE) inhibitors:** ACE inhibitors keep your body from making a hormone called angiotensin II. This hormone normally causes blood vessels to narrow. ACE inhibitors prevent this, so your blood pressure goes down.

- **Angiotensin II receptor blockers:** Angiotensin II receptor blockers (ARBs) are blood pressure medicines that block the effects of angiotensin II. As a result, blood vessels relax and widen, and your blood pressure goes down.

- **Calcium channel blockers:** Calcium channel blockers (CCBs) keep calcium from entering the muscle cells of your heart and blood vessels. This allows blood vessels to relax, and your blood pressure goes down. Some types of CCBs also slow the heart rate.

- **Alpha blockers:** Alpha blockers reduce nerve impulses that tighten blood vessels. This allows blood to flow more freely, causing blood pressure to go down.

- **Alpha-beta blockers:** Alpha-beta blockers reduce nerve impulses the same way alpha blockers do. However, they also slow the heartbeat like beta blockers. As a result, blood pressure goes down.

- **Nervous system inhibitors:** Nervous system inhibitors increase nerve impulses from the brain to relax and widen blood vessels. This causes blood pressure to go down.

- **Vasodilators:** Vasodilators relax the muscles in blood vessel walls. This causes blood pressure to go down.

ACE Inhibitors and Angiotensin Receptor Blockers

Both ACE inhibitors and ARBs relax blood vessels, which lowers blood pressure. Types of ACE inhibitor drugs and ARB drugs are listed in Table 18.1.

Table 18.1. Angiotensin-Converting Enzyme Inhibitors and Angiotensin Receptor Blockers

ACE Inhibitors

Generic Name	Brand Name	Generic Available
Benazepril	Lotensin®	Yes
Captopril	Capoten®	Yes
Enalapril	Vasotec®	Yes
Fosinopril	Monopril®	Yes
Lisinopril	Prinivil®, Zestril®	Yes
Moexipril	Univasc®	No
Perindopril	Aceon®	No
Quinapril	Accupril®	Yes
Ramipril	Altace®	No
Trandolapril	Mavik®	No

ARBs

Generic Name	Brand Name	Generic Available
Candesartan	Atacand®	No
Eprosartan	Teveten®	No
Irbesartan	Avapro®	No
Losartan	Cozaar®	Yes
Olmesartan	Benicar®	No
Telmisartan	Micardis®	No
Valsartan	Diovan®	No

Benefits of ACE Inhibitors and ARBs

It is interesting to compare the benefits of ACE inhibitors and ARBs:

- When taken regularly, both ACE inhibitors and ARBs do a good job of lowering blood pressure. ACE inhibitors and ARBs work equally well.

- They do not affect cholesterol levels or blood sugar levels.

- They rarely cause serious problems.

Which drug is right for you may depend on what you think about the side effects and cost.

Side Effects of ACE Inhibitors and ARBs

Both ACE inhibitors and ARBs can cause cough, dizziness, and headache. The chance of dizziness or headache is about the same with the two drugs. The main difference is that ACE inhibitors are more likely to cause a dry cough. Sometimes this cough is bad enough that people need to switch drugs. Research studies have found that eight out of 100 people taking an ACE inhibitor stop taking it because of side effects and that three out of 100 people taking an ARB stop because of side effects. Tell your doctor or nurse if you are bothered by one of these side effects, but do not stop taking your medicine on your own.

Cost of ACE Inhibitors and ARBs

Cost is often a major factor in using a medicine. If medicines are part of your health insurance plan, check with your plan about the cost to you. Most brand-name ACE inhibitors and ARBs are priced in the range of $75–$125 per month. Many generic ACE inhibitors can be purchased for $4 per month at some pharmacies. Check with your physician regarding which medications are most appropriate for you and with your pharmacy for up-to-date drug prices.

Serious Risks of ACE Inhibitors and ARBs

It is rare, but sometimes people experience a drug reaction called angioedema. In research studies comparing ACE inhibitors and ARBs, about one out of every 10,000 people gets angioedema. Both ACE inhibitors and ARBs can cause angioedema.

The most common symptom of angioedema is swelling of the tongue or lips. Call your doctor or nurse right away if you notice swelling, which might mean you are having a reaction to your medicine.

> **Warning**
>
> If you are taking an ACE inhibitor or an ARB and become pregnant, call your doctor or nurse to ask for advice. ACE inhibitors and ARBs can cause serious birth defects.

ACE Inhibitors and ARBs for the Treatment of Stable Ischemic Heart Disease

According to a new comparative effectiveness review funded by the Agency for Healthcare Research and Quality (AHRQ), treatment featuring ACE inhibitors and ARBs appears to be effective in treating stable ischemic heart disease. Researchers found treatment with the two medications can lead to a reduction in death, a lower risk of heart attack and stroke, and fewer hospitalizations for heart failure for patients suffering from stable ischemic heart disease.

However, these drugs have risks of their own. Risks associated with ACE inhibitors include a persistent cough, sudden fainting, too much potassium in the blood, and dangerously low blood pressure (hypotension). Risks associated with ARBs include too much potassium in the blood and low blood pressure. Knowing the risks and benefits of these medications will help patients and their doctors decide the optimal treatment.

The AHRQ report found that patients with stable ischemic heart disease who take an ACE inhibitor in addition to standard treatment can reduce the likelihood of several negative outcomes, including death from heart attack or heart failure, nonfatal heart attacks, hospitalization for heart failure, and revascularization (surgeries that reroute blood to the heart). Patients who take an ARB in addition to standard medications can reduce their risk of death from a heart-related cause, heart attack, or stroke.

While some patients and clinicians pursue a course of treatment using both ACE inhibitors and ARBs, the report found that combined treatment does not show any benefit over an ACE inhibitor alone and that risks include fainting, diarrhea, low blood pressure, and kidney problems. The report found that existing studies provide few data on the medications' benefits or harms in specific populations such as people of different genders, ethnicity, or diabetic status or those who have or do not have high blood pressure.

Adapted from "High Blood Pressure," National Heart, Lung, and Blood Institute (NHLBI, www.nhlbi.nih.gov), November 2008, and "Comparing Two Kinds of Blood Pressure Pills: ACEIs and ARBs," November 1, 2007, and "High Blood Pressure Medicines Show Promise for Treating Heart Disease," December 2009, both produced by the Agency for Healthcare Research and Quality (AHRQ, www.ahrq.gov).

Chapter 19

Medicines to Manage Blood Cholesterol

When it comes to keeping your heart healthy, the foods you eat and the genes you inherit matter. Good heart health also may depend on the drugs you take. Several medicines are effective at lowering blood cholesterol levels—a key factor in good heart health.

Types of Cholesterol-Lowering Medications

There are five major types of cholesterol-lowering medicines. The different medications each have their own advantages and disadvantages:

- Statins are very effective in lowering low-density lipoprotein (LDL, or bad) cholesterol levels and are safe for most people. Rare side effects to watch for are muscle and liver problems.

- Bile acid sequestrants help lower LDL cholesterol levels and are sometimes prescribed with statins. They are not usually prescribed as the only medicine to lower cholesterol.

- Niacin, or nicotinic acid, lowers LDL cholesterol and triglycerides and raises high-density lipoprotein (HDL, or good) cholesterol. It should be used only under a doctor's supervision.

- Fibrates lower triglycerides and may increase HDL cholesterol levels. When used with a statin, however, they may increase the chance of muscle problems.

- Cholesterol absorption inhibitors, such as ezetimibe, lower LDL cholesterol and act within the intestine to block cholesterol absorption.

Two other types of medications also used to lower cholesterol are omega-3 fatty acids and combination drugs.

When you are under treatment, you will be checked regularly to make sure your cholesterol level is controlled and to check for other health problems.

You may take medicines for other health problems as well. It is important to take all medicines as your doctor prescribes. The combination of medicines may lower your risk for heart disease or heart attack.

Statins

Statins (HMG-CoA reductase inhibitors) are one class of many drugs used to lower the level of cholesterol in the blood by reducing the production of cholesterol by the liver. Statins block the enzyme in the liver responsible for making cholesterol. Too much cholesterol can increase a person's chance of getting heart disease.

Statins are relatively safe for most people, but some can respond differently to the drugs. Certain people may have fewer side effects with one statin drug than another. Some statins, in particular lovastatin and simvastatin, also are known to interact adversely with other drugs. This information, coupled with the degree of cholesterol lowering desired, will help guide the decision about which statin to use or whether another type of drug should be used.

Do All Cholesterol Medications Reduce the Risk of Heart Attack?

There are many medications for high cholesterol on the market. Does it matter which one I take? The answer is not simple.

All the medications discussed in this chapter improve cholesterol levels. It has generally been assumed that improving cholesterol reduces the risk of heart attack. However, evidence is much better for some drugs than others.

Statins are usually the first choices for treatment because of their proven benefits for heart disease. All statins except pitavastatin have been proven to substantially reduce the risk of heart attacks in addition to lowering cholesterol. For this reason, statins are recommended for nearly all patients with coronary artery disease or other very high-risk conditions.

Bile acid sequestrants have also been shown to prevent heart disease in combination with statins. It is unclear to what degree they reduce risk on their own, and they do not appear to be as effective as statins.

With other classes of medications, the situation is less certain. They clearly do improve cholesterol, but it is not as clear whether they reduce the risk of heart disease.

A handful of studies of niacin and gemfibrozil reported they reduce risk of heart disease, at least in some groups of patients. However, other studies have not clearly demonstrated this, and the evidence is not as strong as with statins.

Several studies of fenofibrate have failed to show improvements in heart disease in patients treated with it. However, many patients in these studies were taking statins in combination with fenofibrate, and some researchers argue this obscured the benefits of the drug.

Ezetimibe lowers LDL cholesterol modestly by itself and much more substantially when combined with a statin. However, preliminary studies of a combination of ezetimibe with simvastatin found no reductions in heart disease compared to simvastatin alone, despite achieving much lower LDL cholesterol levels with the combination. A study of niacin versus ezetimibe found that niacin improved a measure of atherosclerosis, but ezetimibe did not. These results have led some researchers to speculate that ezetimibe might have negative effects on the heart that offset its cholesterol-lowering benefits. Studies are underway that will hopefully determine exactly what effect, if any, ezetimibe has on the risk of heart disease.

Types of Statins

The types of statins currently available are as follows:

- Altoprev® (lovastatin)
- Crestor® (rosuvastatin)
- Lescol® (fluvastatin)
- Lipitor® (atorvastatin)
- Livalo® (pitavastatin)
- Mevacor® (lovastatin)
- Pravachol® (pravastatin)
- Zocor® (simvastatin)

Safety Warnings

If you are using statins, there are a few warnings to observe:

- Do not use these medicines if you have liver disease.
- Do not use these medicines if you are pregnant or nursing.
- Use these medicines with caution if you are also taking gemfibrozil, fenofibrates, amiodarone, verapamil, or blood thinners (anticoagulants).
- People who use some HIV medicines, birth control pills (oral contraceptives), nefazodone, or niacin should talk to their doctor about the specific risks of using statins.
- Drinking a quart or more of grapefruit juice every day may affect these statin medicines.

Common Side Effects

Common side effects of statins include gas, dizziness, constipation, headache, diarrhea, and upset stomach.

Call your doctor if you have fever, dark urine, or muscle pain or weakness without a good reason (such as exercise or injury).

Which Statin Should I Take?

Some cardiologists believe one statin is better than another, and drug advertisers each argue their drug is superior. However, the only proven differences among statin medications are the degree of cholesterol lowering, drug interactions, and cost.

For patients with extremely high LDL cholesterol, rosuvastatin, atorvastatin, and simvastatin may be the best choices because their effects at maximum doses are greater than other statins. However, all statins are effective for people with mildly to moderately elevated LDL.

For people who take multiple medications, pravastatin, pitavastatin, and rosuvastatin may be better choices as they are less likely to interact with other drugs.

There are very large differences in cost among statins. Lovastatin, pravastatin, and simvastatin are available generically and may be purchased at some pharmacies for $4 to $10 per month. Rosuvastatin (Crestor), atorvastatin (Lipitor), fluvastatin (Lescol and Lescol XL), and pitavastatin (Livalo) are only available as branded medications and typically cost between $100–150 per month.

Bile Acid Sequestrants

Types of Bile Acid Sequestrants

Types of bile acid sequestrants currently available include the following:

- Colestid® (colestipol)
- LoCholest® oral powder (cholestyramine)
- Prevalite® oral powder (cholestyramine)
- Questran® oral powder (cholestyramine)
- WelChol® (colesevelam)

Safety Warnings

You should be aware of the following warnings if you are using bile acid sequestrants:

- Do not use these drugs if you have problems with your liver or gallbladder.

- People who have bleeding problems, heart disease, stomach ulcers, kidney disease, or an underactive thyroid should talk to their doctor about the risks of taking these medicines.

- People who take spironolactone should talk to their doctor before taking colestipol (Colestid).

Common Side Effects

Common side effects of bile acid sequestrants include heartburn, constipation, gas, indigestion, and nausea.

Call your doctor if you have stomach pain, vomiting, sudden weight loss, or unusual bleeding from your gums or rectum.

Fibrates

Types of Fibrates

Types of fibrates currently available include the following:

- Antara® (fenofibrate)

- Fenoglide® (fenofibrate)

- Lipofen® (fenofibrate)

- Lopid® (gemfibrozil)

- TriCor® (fenofibrate)

- Triglide® (fenofibrate)

- Trilipix® (fenofibric acid)

Safety Warnings

If you are using fibrates, you should be aware of the following safety warnings:

- People with kidney problems, gallbladder disease, or liver disease should not use these drugs.

- Talk to your doctor before taking statins (HMG-CoA reductase inhibitors) to control cholesterol.

- Pregnant women or women who are breastfeeding should talk to their doctor about the risks of taking these drugs.

- People who take diabetes medicines or blood thinners (anticoagulants) should talk to their doctor about the risks of taking these drugs.

Common Side Effects

Common side effects of fibrates include headache, constipation, diarrhea, dizziness, and stomach pain.

Call your doctor if you have muscle pain, weakness, or jaundice (skin or eyes look yellow).

Niacin

Types of Niacin

The types of niacin currently available include the following:

- Niaspan® (niacin)

- Nicotinic acid

Safety Warnings

You need to be aware of the following safety warnings if you are using niacin:

- Do not use niacin if you have liver disease or if you are taking an immediate-release niacin pill.

- Do not use niacin if you are pregnant or breastfeeding.

- People who are taking aspirin, high blood pressure medicines, HMG CoA reductase inhibitors (statins), or medicines to lower bile acid should talk to their doctor about the risks of taking niacin.

- People with kidney disease, peptic ulcer, diabetes, or chest pain should talk to their doctor about the risks of taking this drug.

- People who have had a heart attack or gout should talk to their doctor about the risks of taking this drug.

Common Side Effects

Common side effects of niacin are headache, upset stomach, heartburn, diarrhea, and flushing (redness of the face or neck).

Call your doctor if you have a fast heartbeat, fainting, dizziness, or jaundice.

Cholesterol Absorption Inhibitors

Types of Cholesterol Absorption Inhibitors

The only available prescription cholesterol absorption inhibitor is Zetia® (ezetimibe).

Safety Warnings

If you are taking a cholesterol absorption inhibitor, you need to be aware of the following things:

- Women who are pregnant or breastfeeding should not take Zetia with another cholesterol medicine.

- People who have liver disease should not take Zetia with another cholesterol medicine.

- Use caution if you are taking blood thinners (anticoagulants).

Common Side Effects

Common side effects of Zetia include feeling tired and stomach pain.

Call your doctor if you have muscle pain, tenderness, or weakness; stomach pain; swelling of the face or lips; or severe itching.

Omega-3 Fatty Acids

Types of Omega-3 Fatty Acids

The most commonly prescribed type of omega-3 fatty acid is Lovaza® (omega-3 acid ethyl esters). For information about omega-3 fatty acids available as dietary supplements, see chapter 20.

Safety Warnings

If you are taking an omega-3 fatty acid, you should be aware of the following safety warnings:

- Women who are breastfeeding, pregnant, or planning to become pregnant should talk to their doctor before taking Lovaza.

- Tell your doctor if you have diabetes or liver, thyroid, or pancreas problems.

- Tell your doctor if you are allergic to fish.

- Tell your doctor if you drink more than two glasses of alcohol each day.

- Tell your doctor if you take blood thinners or anticoagulants including aspirin, warfarin, coumarin, and clopidogrel (Plavix®).

Common Side Effects

Common side effects of omega-3 fatty acids include burping, infection, feeling like you have the flu, upset stomach, changes in your sense of taste, back pain, and skin rash. In addition, Lovaza may affect certain blood tests:

- Alanine aminotransferase (ALT) test, which checks your liver

- Low-density lipoprotein cholesterol (LDL-C) test, which checks your cholesterol

Questions to Ask Your Doctor

Here are some questions you might want to ask if your doctor prescribes medication to help control your blood cholesterol:

- What drugs am I taking?
- What are the side effects?
- What other prescription drugs should I avoid while taking my medicines?
- What foods, herbs, or over-the-counter medicines should I avoid?
- When should I take each drug? How many times per day do I take each drug?
- Can I take my medicines if I am pregnant or nursing?

Combination Medicines

Types of Combination Medicines

Types of combination medicines currently available include the following:

- Advicor® (niacin and lovastatin)
- Simcor® (niacin and simvastatin)
- Vytorin® (ezetimibe and simvastatin)

Safety Warnings

If you are taking a combination medicine, you need to be aware of the following warnings:

- Do not take Vytorin, Simcor, or Advicor if you are pregnant or breastfeeding.
- Do not take Vytorin if you have liver disease.

- People taking gemfibrozil (Lopid), fenofibrate (TriCor), high blood pressure medicines, protease inhibitors (medicines to treat HIV), or blood thinners (anticoagulants) should use caution when taking these drugs.

- Drinking a quart or more of grapefruit juice every day may affect these drugs.

Common Side Effects

Common side effects of combination medicines for controlling blood cholesterol include headache, flushing (redness of the face or neck), and upset stomach.

Call your doctor if you have dark urine; stomach pain; muscle pain, tenderness, or weakness without a good reason (such as exercise or injury); or jaundice.

Other Combination Medicines

Another type of combination medicine used to control blood cholesterol is Caduet®, which combines amlodipine and atorvastatin. Caduet is used to treat people who have both high blood pressure and high cholesterol.

Safety Warnings

Things to be aware of if you are taking Caduet include the following:

- Do not take Caduet if you are pregnant or planning to become pregnant.

- Do not take Caduet if you are breastfeeding.

- Do not take Caduet if you have liver problems.

Common Side Effects

Common side effects of Caduet include swelling of the legs or ankles (edema), muscle or joint pain, headache, diarrhea, constipation, feeling dizzy, feeling tired or sleepy, gas, rash, nausea, stomach pain, fast or irregular heartbeat, and face feeling hot or warm (flushing).

Call your doctor if you have muscle problems like weakness, tenderness, or pain without a good reason (such as exercise or injury); brown or dark-colored urine; jaundice; or more tiredness than usual.

Adapted from "High Blood Cholesterol," National Heart, Lung, and Blood Institute (NHLBI, www.nhlbi.nih.gov), September 2008, and "High Cholesterol— Medicines to Help You," August 2009, and "Controlling Cholesterol with Statins," February 22, 2010, both produced by the U.S. Food and Drug Administration (FDA, www.fda.gov), with supplemental information added by David A. Cooke, MD, FACP, April 2010.

Chapter 20

Dietary Supplements

There are a number of dietary supplements used for the treatment of high cholesterol and heart disease. The effectiveness of these supplements is for the most part unproven, and some research studies seem to indicate they are, in fact, not effective at all. This chapter examines the current evidence on the effectiveness of some of the most commonly used dietary supplements in the treatment of high cholesterol and heart disease.

Omega-3 Fatty Acids

Since the first studies in the 1970s, the evidence supporting a role for omega-3 fatty acids in the prevention of cardiovascular disease (CVD) has continued to increase. However, the beneficial effects of omega-3 fatty acids are not consistently observed in all studies.

The Agency for Healthcare Research and Quality recently undertook a review of information from experimental and observational studies that investigated the effect of dietary or supplemental omega-3 fatty acids on clinical outcomes. More specifically, they examined how dietary or supplemental omega-3 fatty acids affect particular cardiovascular disease outcomes such as heart attack and stroke and investigated whether omega-3 fatty acids can play a role in primary and secondary prevention of these outcomes. In addition, they examined evidence of adverse events and drug interactions associated with omega-3 fatty acids.

Effects of Omega-3 Fatty Acid Supplements or Fish Consumption on Cardiovascular Disease Outcomes

A number of studies were analyzed. All these studies quantified or estimated the intake of fish or omega-3 fatty acids and assessed the effects of their consumption on CVD outcomes.

Overall, the evidence supports the hypothesis that consumption of omega-3 fatty acids, fish, and fish oil reduces all-cause mortality and various CVD outcomes such as sudden death, cardiac death (coronary or myocardial infarction death), and myocardial infarction, although the evidence is strongest for fish or fish oil. The relative effect of omega-3 fatty acids on stroke is uncertain.

Furthermore, these studies found no consistent difference in the effect of omega-3 fatty acids on CVD outcomes between men and women, though a report based on the first National Health and Nutrition Examination that separately analyzed data for men and women found a trend of decreased stroke with increasing fish consumption for women between ages 45 and 74, but not for men.

Adverse Events Associated with Omega-3 Fatty Acid Consumption

A total of 142 studies were reviewed to determine the severity of adverse events associated with the consumption of omega-3 fatty acids. None of the studies associated omega-3 fatty acid consumption with events such as death, life-threatening illness, or significant disability or handicap, although two studies reported some important bleeding with fish oil combined with aspirin or warfarin.

Flaxseed and Flaxseed Oil

Flaxseed (common name: flaxseed, linseed; Latin name; *Linum usitatissimum*) is the seed of the flax plant, which is believed to have originated in Egypt. It grows throughout Canada and the northwestern United States. Flaxseed oil comes from flaxseeds. Both flaxseed and flaxseed oil have been used for high cholesterol levels and in an effort to prevent cancer.

How Flaxseed Is Used

Whole or crushed flaxseed can be mixed with water or juice and taken by mouth. Flaxseed is also available in powder form. Flaxseed oil is available in liquid and capsule form. Flaxseed contains lignans (phytoestrogens, or plant estrogens), while flaxseed oil preparations lack lignans.

What the Science Says

Results are mixed in research studies to date on the effectiveness of flaxseed for medicinal purposes:

- Flaxseed contains soluble fiber, like that found in oat bran, and has been found to be an effective laxative.

- Studies of flaxseed preparations to lower cholesterol levels report mixed results.

- Some studies suggest that alpha-linolenic acid (a substance found in flaxseed and flaxseed oil) may benefit people with heart disease. But not enough reliable data are available to determine whether flaxseed is effective for heart conditions.

- Study results are mixed on whether flaxseed decreases hot flashes.

- The National Center for Complementary and Alternative Medicine (NCCAM) is funding studies on flaxseed. Recent studies have looked at the effects of flaxseed on high cholesterol levels, as well as its possible role in preventing conditions such as heart disease and osteoporosis.

Side Effects and Cautions

Flaxseed and flaxseed oil supplements seem to be well tolerated. Few side effects have been reported.

Flaxseed, like any supplemental fiber source, should be taken with plenty of water; otherwise, it could worsen constipation or, in rare cases, even cause intestinal blockage.

The fiber in flaxseed may lower the body's ability to absorb medications taken by mouth. Flaxseed should not be taken at the same time as any conventional oral medications or other dietary supplements.

Tell your health care providers about any complementary and alternative practices you use. Give them a full picture of what you do to manage your health. This will help ensure coordinated and safe care.

Garlic

A recent study from Stanford University has cast doubt on the effectiveness of garlic to lower LDL cholesterol levels in adults with moderately high cholesterol. LDL cholesterol is widely known as bad cholesterol and is believed to be a leading contributor to heart disease.

Christopher Gardner, PhD, and colleagues conducted a randomized, placebo-controlled trial studying whether three different formulations of garlic could lower LDL cholesterol. The study participants were randomly divided into four groups that received raw garlic, a powdered garlic supplement, an aged extract supplement, or a placebo.

The 169 participants who completed the study had their cholesterol levels checked monthly for the duration of the six-month trial. None of the formulations of garlic had a statistically significant effect on LDL cholesterol levels.

The authors caution that these results should not be generalized for all populations or all health effects. An accompanying editorial in the journal *Archives of Internal Medicine* points out that LDL cholesterol levels are only one factor contributing to heart disease and that this trial did not investigate garlic's effects on other risk factors, such as high blood pressure.

Hawthorn

Hawthorn (common names: hawthorn, English hawthorn, harthorne, haw, hawthorne; Latin names: *Crataegus laevigata,* also known as *Crataegus oxyacantha, Crataegus monogyna*) is a spiny, flowering shrub or small tree of the rose family. The species of hawthorn discussed here are native to northern European regions and grow throughout the world.

Recently, hawthorn leaf and flower have been used for heart failure. Hawthorn is also used for other heart conditions, including symptoms of coronary artery disease (such as angina).

How Hawthorn Is Used

The hawthorn leaf and flower are used to make liquid extracts, usually with water and alcohol. Dry extracts can be put into capsules and tablets.

What the Science Says

There is limited scientific evidence that hawthorn leaf and flower are safe and effective for milder forms of heart failure. It is not clear how treatment with hawthorn compares to other medications for heart failure. There is not enough scientific evidence to determine whether hawthorn works for other heart problems. NCCAM-supported research to date includes a study of the mechanism by which hawthorn may affect heart failure.

Side Effects and Cautions

Hawthorn is considered safe for most adults when used for short periods of time. Side effects are usually mild and can include upset stomach, headache, and dizziness.

Drug interactions with hawthorn have not been thoroughly studied. It was once thought hawthorn interacted with the heart medicine digoxin. However, a very small study in people without heart conditions found no interaction, but evidence is limited.

Tell your health care providers about any complementary and alternative practices you use. Give them a full picture of what you do to manage your health. This will help ensure coordinated and safe care.

Adapted from "Effects of Omega-3 Fatty Acids on Cardiovascular Disease," Agency for Healthcare Research and Quality (AHRQ, www.ahrq.gov), undated, and "Flaxseed and Flaxseed Oil," April 2008, "Garlic Does Not Appear to Lower 'Bad' Cholesterol," undated, and "Hawthorn," May 2008, all three produced by the National Center for Complementary and Alternative Medicine (NCCAM, www.nccam.nih.gov).

Chapter 21

Heart Surgery

Heart surgery is done to correct problems with the heart. More than half a million heart surgeries are done each year in the United States for a variety of heart problems.

Traditional heart surgery, often called open-heart surgery, is done by opening the chest wall to operate on the heart. The chest is almost always opened by cutting through a patient's breastbone. Once the heart is exposed, the patient is connected to a heart-lung bypass machine. The machine takes over the pumping action of the heart, which allows surgeons to operate on a still heart.

Other methods of heart surgery also have been developed. One way is called off-pump, or beating heart, surgery. It's like traditional open-heart surgery, but it doesn't use a heart-lung bypass machine.

Another type of surgery, called minimally invasive heart surgery, uses smaller incisions (cuts) than traditional open-heart surgery. Some types of minimally invasive heart surgery use a heart-lung bypass machine and others don't.

These nontraditional methods may reduce risks and speed recovery time. Studies are underway to compare these types of heart surgery with traditional open-heart surgery. The results of these studies will help doctors decide the best procedure to use for each patient.

The results of heart surgery in adults often are excellent. Heart surgery can reduce symptoms, improve quality of life, and increase lifespan.

Types of Heart Surgery

Various types of heart surgery are used to fix various heart problems.

Coronary Artery Bypass Grafting

Coronary artery bypass grafting (CABG) is the most common type of heart surgery. More than 500,000 of these surgeries are done each year in the United States. CABG improves blood flow to the heart. This surgery is used for people who have severe coronary heart disease (CHD), also called coronary artery disease. CABG is discussed in chapter 23.

Transmyocardial Laser Revascularization

Transmyocardial laser revascularization, or TLR, is a surgery used to treat angina when no other treatments work. For example, if you've already had one CABG procedure and can't have another one, TLR may be an option. This type of heart surgery isn't common.

During TLR, a surgeon uses lasers to make channels in the heart muscle. These channels allow oxygen-rich blood to flow from a heart chamber directly into the heart muscle.

Heart Valve Repair or Replacement

For the heart to work right, blood must flow in only one direction. The heart's valves make this possible. Healthy valves open and close in a precise way as the heart pumps blood.

Each valve has a set of flaps called leaflets. The leaflets open to allow blood to pass from the heart chambers into the arteries. Then the leaflets close tightly to stop blood from flowing back into the chambers.

Heart surgery is done to fix leaflets that don't open as wide as they should, which can happen if they become thick, stiff, or fused together. As a result, not enough blood flows through the valve into the artery.

Heart surgery also is done to fix leaflets that don't close tightly. If leaflets don't close tightly, blood can leak backward into the heart chambers rather than moving only forward into the arteries as it should.

To fix these problems, surgeons either repair the valve or replace it. Replacement valves are taken from animals or made from human tissue or man-made materials.

To repair a mitral or pulmonary valve that's too narrow, a surgeon will insert a catheter (a thin, flexible tube) through a large blood vessel and guide it to the heart. This procedure is called cardiac catheterization. The surgeon will place the end of the catheter inside the narrowed valve. He or she will rapidly inflate and deflate a small balloon at the tip of the catheter. This widens the valve, allowing blood to flow through it to the artery. This approach is less invasive than open-heart surgery.

Researchers also are testing new ways to use catheters in other types of valve surgeries. For example, catheters may be used to place clips on the mitral valve leaflets to hold them in place or to replace a valve that doesn't work well.

Only a few medical centers are doing these experimental procedures. However, the results may lead to improved heart surgery approaches.

Arrhythmia Treatment

Arrhythmias usually are treated with medicine first. If medicine doesn't work well enough, you may need surgery. For example, your doctor may use surgery to implant a pacemaker or an implantable cardioverter defibrillator (ICD). ICDs are discussed in chapter 24, and pacemakers are discussed in chapter 25.

Another type of surgery for arrhythmia is called maze surgery. In this operation, the surgeon makes new paths for the heart's electrical signals to travel through. This type of surgery is used to treat atrial fibrillation, the most common type of serious arrhythmia.

Simpler, less invasive procedures also are used to treat atrial fibrillation. These procedures use high heat or intense cold to prevent abnormal electrical signals from moving through the heart, which helps the heart's electrical signals move through the proper pathway.

Aneurysm Repair

An aneurysm is an abnormal bulge or ballooning in the wall of an artery or the heart muscle. Over time, an aneurysm can grow and burst, causing dangerous, often fatal bleeding inside the body.

Aneurysms in the heart most often occur in the heart's lower left chamber (the left ventricle). Repairing an aneurysm involves surgery to replace the weak section of the artery or heart wall with a patch or graft.

Heart Transplant

A heart transplant is surgery to remove a person's diseased heart and replace it with a healthy heart from a deceased donor. Your doctor may recommend a heart transplant if your heart is so damaged or weak it can't pump enough blood to meet your body's needs. Heart transplants are discussed in chapter 26.

Ventricular Assist Devices

Ventricular assist devices (VADs) are mechanical pumps used to support heart function and blood flow in people who have weakened hearts. Your doctor may recommend a VAD if you have heart failure or if you're waiting for a heart transplant. You can use a VAD for a short time or for months or years, depending on your situation.

Surgical Approaches

Depending on a patient's heart problem, general health, and other factors, he or she can have open-heart surgery or minimally invasive heart surgery.

Open-Heart Surgery

Open-heart surgery is any kind of surgery in which a surgeon makes a large incision in the chest to open the rib cage and operate on the heart. *Open* refers to the chest, not the heart. Depending on the type of surgery, the surgeon also may open the heart.

Open-heart surgery is used to bypass blocked arteries in the heart, repair or replace heart valves, treat atrial fibrillation, and do heart transplants.

Increasing numbers of surgeons have started to use off-pump, or beating heart, surgery to do CABG. This approach is like traditional open-heart surgery, but surgeons don't use a heart-lung bypass machine. However, it is not clear that off-pump surgery is better than traditional procedures. A study published in 2009 in the *New England Journal of Medicine* found worse outcomes in patients who had off-pump surgery.

Off-pump heart surgery isn't right for all patients. Work with your doctor to decide whether this type of surgery may benefit you. Your doctor will carefully consider your heart problem, age, overall health, and other factors that may affect the surgery.

Minimally Invasive Heart Surgery

In minimally invasive heart surgery, a surgeon makes small incisions in the side of the chest between the ribs. A heart-lung bypass machine is used for some types of minimally invasive heart surgery.

Minimally invasive heart surgery is used for some CABG and maze procedures. It's also used to repair or replace heart valves and insert pacemakers or ICDs.

One type of minimally invasive heart surgery that's still being developed is robotic-assisted surgery. For this surgery, a surgeon uses a computer to control surgical tools on thin robotic arms.

The tools are inserted through small incisions in the chest, which allows the surgeon to do complex and highly precise surgery. The surgeon always is in total control of the robotic arms; they don't move on their own.

When Heart Surgery Is Necessary

Heart surgery is used to treat people who have certain heart diseases and conditions. If other treatments—such as lifestyle changes, medicine, and medical procedures—haven't worked or can't be used, heart surgery may be an option.

Heart surgery is used to treat heart failure and coronary heart disease. It's also used to fix heart valves that don't work right, control heart rhythms, and replace damaged hearts with healthy ones.

Specialists Involved

Your primary care doctor, a cardiologist, and a cardiothoracic surgeon will work with you to decide whether you need heart surgery. A cardiologist specializes in diagnosing and treating heart problems. A cardiothoracic surgeon specializes in surgery on the heart and lungs.

These doctors will talk with you and do tests to learn about your general health and your heart problem. They'll discuss test results with you, and you'll help make decisions about the surgery.

What to Expect before Heart Surgery

There are many types of heart surgery. The type you need depends on your situation. One person's experience before surgery can be very different from another's.

Some people carefully plan their surgeries with their doctors. They know exactly when and how their surgeries will happen. Other people need emergency heart surgery. Others are diagnosed with blocked coronary arteries and are admitted to the hospital right away for surgery as soon as possible.

If you're having a planned surgery, you may be admitted to the hospital the afternoon or morning before your surgery. Your doctors and others on your health care team will meet with you to explain what will happen. They'll give you instructions on how to prepare for the surgery.

You also may need to have some tests, such as an EKG, chest x-ray, or blood tests. An IV line will be placed into a blood vessel in your arm or chest to give you fluids and medicines.

Hair near the incision site may be shaved. Your skin may be washed with special soap to reduce the risk of infection.

Just before the surgery, you'll be moved to the operating room. You'll be given medicine to make you fall asleep and feel no pain during the surgery.

What to Expect during Heart Surgery

Heart surgery is done in a hospital. A team of experts is involved. Cardiothoracic surgeons perform the surgery assisted by a team of other doctors and nurses. The length of time for the surgery depends on the type of surgery. CABG, the most common type of heart surgery, usually takes three to five hours.

Traditional Open-Heart Surgery

For this type of surgery, you're given medicine to make you fall asleep. A doctor checks your heartbeat, blood pressure, oxygen levels, and breathing during the surgery. A breathing tube is placed in your lungs through your throat and connected to a ventilator (breathing machine).

A surgeon makes a 6- to 8-inch incision (cut) down the center of your chest wall. Your breastbone is cut and your rib cage opened so the surgeon can get to your heart.

You're given medicine to thin your blood and keep it from clotting. A heart-lung bypass machine is connected to your heart. This machine takes over for your heart by replacing its pumping action. A specialist oversees the machine. The bypass machine allows the surgeon to operate on a heart that isn't moving and full of blood.

You're given medicines to stop your heartbeat once you're connected to the heart-lung bypass machine. A tube is placed in your heart to drain blood to the machine. The machine removes carbon dioxide (a waste product) from your blood, adds oxygen, and then pumps the blood back into your body. Tubes are inserted into your chest to drain fluid. Once the bypass machine begins to work, the surgeon begins the surgery to repair your heart problem.

After the surgery is completed, blood flow to your heart is restored. Usually the heart starts beating again on its own. In some cases, mild electric shocks are used to restart the heart. Once the heart has started beating again, the tubes are removed and the heart-lung bypass machine is stopped. You're given medicine to allow your blood to clot again.

The surgeon uses wires to close your breastbone. The wires stay in your body permanently. After your breastbone heals, it will be as strong as it was before the surgery.

Stitches or staples are used to close the skin incision, and the breathing tube is removed when you're able to breathe without it.

Off-Pump Heart Surgery

This type of surgery is the same as traditional open-heart surgery except you aren't connected to a heart-lung bypass machine. Instead, your heart is steadied with a mechanical device while the surgeon works on it. Your heart continues to pump blood to your body.

Minimally Invasive Heart Surgery

For this type of heart surgery, the surgeon makes small incisions in the side of your chest between the ribs. These incisions can be as small as 2 to 3 inches. Then the surgeon inserts surgical tools through these small incisions.

A tool with a small video camera at the tip also is inserted through an incision, which allows the surgeon to see inside the body. Some types of minimally invasive heart surgery use a heart-lung bypass machine; other types don't.

What to Expect after Heart Surgery

Recovery in the Hospital

Depending on the type of heart surgery, you may spend a day or more in the hospital's intensive care unit (ICU). You may have an IV needle inserted in a blood vessel in your arm or chest to give you fluids until you're ready to drink on your own.

You also may be given extra oxygen through a face mask or nasal prongs that fit just inside your nose. These pieces of equipment are removed when you no longer need them.

When you leave the ICU, you'll be moved to another part of the hospital for several days before you go home. The entire time you're at the hospital, doctors and nurses will closely watch your heart rate, blood pressure, breathing, vital signs, and incision site(s).

Recovery at Home

Each person responds differently to heart surgery. Your recovery at home will depend on what kind of heart problem and surgery you had. Your doctor will give you specific instructions about how to care for your healing incisions, recognize signs of infection or other complications, and cope with aftereffects of surgery. You also will receive information about follow-up appointments, medicines, and situations when you should call your doctor right away.

Aftereffects of heart surgery are normal. They may include muscle pain, chest pain, or swelling (especially if you have an incision in your leg from CABG). Other aftereffects may include loss of appetite, problems sleeping, constipation, and mood swings and depression. Aftereffects usually go away over time.

Recovery time varies for different types of heart surgery. Full recovery from traditional open-heart CABG may take 6 to 12 weeks or more. Less recovery time is needed for off-pump heart surgery and minimally invasive heart surgery.

Your doctor will let you know when you can go back to your daily activities, such as working, driving, and physical activity.

Ongoing Care

Care after your surgery may include periodic checkups with your doctor. During these visits, you may have blood tests, an EKG, echocardiography, or a stress test. These tests will show how your heart is working after the surgery.

Your doctor also may talk with you about lifestyle changes and medicines to help you stay healthy. Lifestyle changes may include quitting smoking, making changes to your diet, engaging in regular physical activity, and reducing and managing stress.

You doctor may refer you to a cardiac rehabilitation (rehab) program. Cardiac rehab includes counseling, education, and exercise training to help you recover. The program also will help you learn how to make choices that can lower your risk of future heart problems.

Risks of Heart Surgery

Heart surgery has risks, even though its results are often excellent. Risks include bleeding and infection, fever, swelling, and other signs of inflammation. Reactions to the medicine used to temporarily put you to sleep during surgery are another risk. Some people may experience arrhythmias (irregular heartbeats), memory loss and problems concentrating or thinking clearly, or damage to tissues in the heart, kidneys, and lungs.

The use of a heart-lung bypass machine increases the risk of blood clots forming in your blood vessels. Clots can travel to the brain or other parts of the body and block the flow of blood. This can cause stroke or other problems. Improvements in heart-lung bypass machines and heart surgery techniques are helping reduce the risk of blood clots.

And, unfortunately, some people die. Heart surgery is more likely to be life threatening in people who are very sick before the surgery. In general, the risks of heart surgery are higher for people who are older than 70, have had previous heart surgeries, or have diseases or conditions such as high blood pressure, diabetes, kidney disease, lung disease, or peripheral arterial disease.

Adapted from "Heart Surgery," National Heart, Lung, and Blood Institute (NHLBI, www.nhlbi.nih.gov), February 2010.

Chapter 22

Angioplasty

Coronary angioplasty is a procedure used to open blocked or narrowed coronary arteries. Coronary angioplasty is also known by other names, including percutaneous coronary intervention and balloon angioplasty.

When Coronary Angioplasty Is Necessary

Angioplasty is one of a number of treatments for coronary heart disease. Other treatments include medicines and coronary artery bypass grafting (CABG). Your doctor will consider many factors when deciding what treatment or combination of treatments to recommend. Compared with CABG, there are some advantages to angioplasty: it doesn't require an incision, it doesn't require general anesthesia (that is, you won't be temporarily put to sleep during the procedure), and it has a shorter recovery time.

Angioplasty also is used as an emergency procedure during a heart attack. As plaque builds up in the coronary arteries, it can rupture. This can cause a blood clot to form on the plaque's surface and block blood flow. Quickly opening a blockage lessens the damage during a heart attack by restoring blood flow to the heart muscle. Angioplasty usually is the fastest way to open a blocked artery and is the best approach during a heart attack.

A disadvantage of angioplasty, when compared with CABG, is that the artery more frequently renarrows over time. The risk of this happening is lower when stents are used, especially stents coated with medicine (drug-eluting stents). However, stents aren't without risks. In some cases, blood clots can form in stents and cause a heart attack.

Your doctor will talk to you about your treatment options and which procedure is best for you.

How Coronary Angioplasty Is Done

Before your coronary angioplasty, your doctor will need to know the location and extent of the blockages in your coronary arteries. To find this information, your doctor will use coronary angiography. This procedure, which was discussed in chapter 14, uses a small tube called a catheter and a special dye that can be seen on an x-ray. X-ray pictures are taken as the dye flows through your coronary arteries to tell your doctor the location and extent of the blockages.

For the angioplasty procedure, another catheter with a balloon on its tip (called a balloon catheter) is inserted in the coronary artery and positioned in the blockage. The balloon is then expanded pushing the plaque against the artery wall and relieving the blockage and improving blood flow.

A small mesh tube called a stent usually is placed in the artery during angioplasty. The stent supports the inner artery wall and reduces the chance of the artery becoming narrowed or blocked again.

Some stents are coated with medicine that is slowly and continuously released into the artery. These are called drug-eluting stents. The medicine helps prevent the artery from becoming blocked with scar tissue growing in the artery.

What to Expect before Coronary Angioplasty

Cardiologists perform coronary angioplasties at hospitals. If your angioplasty isn't done as an emergency treatment, you'll meet with your cardiologist before the procedure. He or she will go over your medical history (including the medicines you take), do a physical exam, and talk to you about the procedure. Your doctor also may recommend some routine tests, such as blood tests, an EKG, and a chest x-ray.

Once the angioplasty is scheduled, your doctor will advise you about when to begin fasting (not eating or drinking) before the procedure. Often you have to stop eating and drinking by midnight the night before the procedure. You doctor will also tell you what medicines you should and shouldn't take on the day of the angioplasty, when to arrive at the hospital, and where to go.

Even though angioplasty takes only one to two hours, you'll likely need to stay in the hospital overnight or longer. Your doctor may advise you not to drive for a certain amount of time after the procedure, so you may have to arrange for a ride home.

What to Expect during Coronary Angioplasty

Coronary angioplasty is done in a special part of the hospital called the cardiac catheterization laboratory. The cath lab has special video screens and x-ray machines. Your doctor uses this equipment to see enlarged pictures of the blockages in your coronary arteries.

Preparation

In the cath lab, you'll lie on a table. An IV line will be placed in your arm to give you fluids and medicine. The medicine will relax you and prevent blood clots from forming.

In preparation for the procedure, the area where your doctor will insert the catheter will be shaved. The catheter usually is inserted in your groin (upper thigh). The shaved area will be cleaned and then numbed. The numbing medicine may sting as it's going in.

The Procedure

During angioplasty, you'll be awake but sleepy.

Your doctor will use a needle to make a small hole in an artery in your arm or groin. A thin, flexible guide wire will be inserted into the artery through the small hole. The needle will then be removed, and a tapered tube called a sheath will be placed over the guide wire and into the artery.

Next, your doctor will put a long, thin, flexible tube called a guiding catheter through the sheath and slide it over the guide wire. The catheter will be moved to the opening of a coronary artery, and the guide wire will be removed.

Next, your doctor will inject a small amount of special dye through the catheter. This will help show the inside of the coronary artery and any blockages on an x-ray picture called an angiogram.

Another guide wire will then be put through the catheter into the coronary artery and threaded past the blockage. The balloon catheter will be threaded over the wire and through the guiding catheter. Then it will be positioned in the blockage. The balloon will then be inflated, which will push the plaque against the artery wall, relieving the blockage and improving blood flow through the artery. Sometimes the balloon will be inflated and deflated more than once to widen the artery. Afterward, the balloon catheter, guiding catheter, and guide wire will be removed.

A drill-like device called a rotablator sometimes is used to remove very hard plaque from the artery.

Your doctor may put a stent (small mesh tube) in your artery to help keep it open. If so, the stent will be wrapped around the balloon catheter. When your doctor inflates the balloon, the stent will expand against the wall of the artery. When the balloon is deflated and pulled out of the artery with the catheter, the stent will remain in place in the artery.

After the angioplasty is complete, the hole in your artery where the sheath, guide wires, and catheters were inserted will be sealed with a special device, or pressure will be put on it until the blood vessel seals.

During angioplasty, strong anticlotting medicine will be given through the IV line to prevent blood clots from forming in the artery or on the stent. This medicine makes it less likely your blood will clot. Some anticlotting medicines may be started before the angioplasty.

What to Expect after Coronary Angioplasty

After coronary angioplasty, you'll be moved to a special care unit. You'll stay there for a few hours or overnight. You must lie still for a few hours to allow the blood vessel in your arm or groin (upper thigh) to seal completely.

While you recover, nurses will check your heart rate and blood pressure. They also will check your arm or groin for bleeding. After a few hours, you'll be able to walk with help.

The place where the catheters (tubes) were inserted may feel sore or tender for about a week.

Going Home

Most people go home the day after the procedure. When your doctor thinks you're ready to leave the hospital, you'll get instructions to follow at home, including how much activity or exercise you can do, when you should follow up with your doctor, and what medicines you should take. Your instructions will also tell you what to look for daily when checking for signs of infection around the area where the tube was inserted. Signs of infection may include redness, swelling, or drainage. You will be told when you should call your doctor. For example, you may need to call if you have shortness of breath, a fever, or signs of infection, pain, or bleeding where the tubes were inserted. You will also be told when you should call 911 (for example, if you have any chest pain).

Your doctor will prescribe medicine to prevent blood clots from forming. Taking your medicine as directed is very important. If you received a stent during angioplasty, the medicine reduces the risk blood clots will form in the stent. Blood clots in the stent can block blood flow and cause a heart attack.

Recovery and Recuperation

Most people recover from angioplasty and return to work about one week after leaving the hospital. Your doctor will want to check your progress after you leave the hospital. During the follow-up visit, your doctor will examine you, make changes to your medicines (if needed), do any necessary tests, and check your overall recovery.

Use this time to ask questions you may have about activities, medicines, or lifestyle changes or to talk about any other issues that concern you.

Risks of Coronary Angioplasty

Coronary angioplasty is a common medical procedure. Serious complications don't occur often. However, they can happen no matter how careful your doctor is or how well he or she does the procedure. Serious complications include bleeding from the blood vessel where the catheters were inserted, blood vessel damage from the catheters, and an allergic reaction to the dye given during the angioplasty. Some people may also experience an arrhythmia (irregular heartbeat).

If an artery closes down instead of opening up, there may be a need for emergency coronary artery bypass grafting during the procedure. This occurs in approximately 2 to 4% of people undergoing angioplasty. CABG is discussed in chapter 23.

Other risks include damage to the kidneys caused by the dye used, heart attack (which occurs in 3 to 5% of people undergoing angioplasty), or stroke (which occurs in less than 1% of people).

Sometimes chest pain can occur during angioplasty because the balloon briefly blocks blood supply to the heart.

As with any procedure involving the heart, complications can sometimes, though rarely, cause death. Less than 2% of people die during angioplasty. The risk of complications is higher in people aged 75 and older, people who have kidney disease or diabetes, women, people who have poor pumping function in their hearts, and people who have extensive heart disease and blockages in their coronary arteries.

Research on angioplasty is ongoing to make it safer and more effective, to prevent treated arteries from closing again, and to make the procedure an option for more people.

Complications from Stents

Restenosis

After angioplasty, the treated coronary artery can become narrowed or blocked again—often within six months of angioplasty. This is called restenosis. When a stent (small mesh tube) isn't used during angioplasty, 4 out of 10 people have restenosis.

The growth of scar tissue in and around a stent also can cause restenosis. When a stent is used, 2 out of 10 people have restenosis.

Stents coated with medicine reduce the growth of scar tissue around the stent and lower the chance of restenosis even more. When these stents are used, about 1 in 10 people has restenosis.

Other treatments, such as radiation, can help prevent tissue growth within a stent. For this procedure, a wire is put through a catheter to where the stent is placed. The wire releases radiation to stop any tissue growth that may block the artery.

Blood Clots

Studies suggest there's a higher risk of blood clots forming in medicine-coated stents compared to bare metal stents. However, no conclusive evidence shows these stents increase the chances of having a heart attack or dying if used as recommended.

When medicine-coated stents are used in people who have advanced CHD, there is a higher risk of blood clots, heart attack, and death. Researchers continue to study medicine-coated stents, including their use in people who have advanced CHD.

Taking medicine as prescribed by your doctor can lower your risk of blood clots. People who have medicine-coated stents usually are advised to take anticlotting medicines, such as clopidogrel and aspirin, for months to years to lower the risk of blood clots.

As with all procedures, it's important to talk with your doctor about your treatment options, including the risks and benefits.

Excerpted and adapted from "Coronary Angioplasty," National Heart, Lung, and Blood Institute (NHLBI, www.nhlbi.nih.gov), January 2010.

Chapter 23

Bypass Surgery

Coronary artery bypass grafting (CABG) is a type of surgery that improves blood flow to the heart. It's used for people who have severe coronary heart disease (CHD), also called coronary artery disease (CAD). CABG is known by several names, including bypass surgery, coronary artery bypass surgery, and heart bypass surgery.

During CABG, a healthy artery or vein from the body is connected, or grafted, to the blocked coronary artery. The grafted artery or vein bypasses (that is, goes around) the blocked portion of the coronary artery. This creates a new passage, and oxygen-rich blood is routed around the blockage to the heart muscle. As many as four major blocked coronary arteries can be bypassed during one surgery.

Types of Coronary Artery Bypass Grafting

Traditional CABG

This is the most common type of CABG. It's used when at least one major artery needs to be bypassed.

During the surgery, the chest bone is opened to access the heart. Medicine is given to stop the heart, and a heart-lung bypass machine is used to keep blood and oxygen moving throughout the body during surgery, allowing the surgeon to operate on a still heart.

After surgery, blood flow to the heart is restored. Usually the heart starts beating again on its own. In some cases, mild electric shocks are used to restart the heart.

Off-Pump CABG

This type of CABG is similar to traditional CABG because the chest bone is opened to access the heart. However, the heart isn't stopped, and a heart-lung bypass machine isn't used. Off-pump CABG is sometimes called beating heart bypass grafting.

Minimally Invasive Direct CABG

This surgery is similar to off-pump CABG. However, instead of a large incision to open the chest bone, several small incisions are made on the left side of the chest between the ribs. This type of surgery mainly is used for bypassing the blood vessels in front of the heart. It's a fairly new procedure that's done less often than the other types of CABG.

This type of CABG isn't for everybody, especially if more than one or two coronary arteries need to be bypassed.

When Coronary Artery Bypass Grafting Is Necessary

CABG is used to treat people who have severe CHD that could lead to a heart attack. CABG also may be used to treat people who have heart damage following a heart attack but still have blocked arteries.

Your doctor may recommend CABG if other treatments, such as lifestyle changes or medicine, haven't worked. He or she also may recommend CABG if you have severe blockages in the large coronary arteries that supply a major part of the heart muscle with blood—especially if your heart's pumping action has already been weakened.

Studies have indicated that patients with diabetes tend to do better over time when treated with CABG than angioplasty. CABG is, therefore, generally preferred for diabetics, but decisions are made on an individual basis.

CABG also may be a treatment option if you have blockages in the heart that can't be treated with angioplasty.

Your doctor will decide whether you're a candidate for CABG based on a number of factors, including the presence and severity of CHD symptoms, the severity and location of blockages in your coronary arteries, your response to other treatments, your quality of life, and any other medical problems you have.

CABG may be done on an emergency basis, such as during a heart attack.

Physical Exam and Diagnostic Tests

To decide whether you're a candidate for CABG, your doctor will do a physical exam. He or she will check your cardiovascular system, focusing on your heart, lungs, and pulse.

Your doctor also will ask you about any symptoms you have, such as chest pain or shortness of breath. He or she will want to know how often and for how long your symptoms occur and how severe they are.

Tests will be done to find out which arteries are clogged, how much they're clogged, and whether there's any heart damage. These tests may include EKG, stress test, echocardiography, and coronary angiography.

Other Considerations

When deciding whether you're a candidate for CABG, your doctor also will consider your history and past treatment of heart disease, including surgeries, procedures, and medicines. Additionally, your doctor will take into account your history of other diseases and conditions, your age and general health, and your family history of CHD, heart attack, or other heart diseases.

Medicines and other medical procedures may be tried before CABG. Medicines that lower cholesterol levels and blood pressure and improve blood flow through the coronary arteries often are tried. Angioplasty, which was described in chapter 22, also may be tried.

What to Expect before Coronary Artery Bypass Grafting

Tests may be done to prepare you for CABG. For example, you may have blood tests, an EKG, echocardiography, a chest x-ray, cardiac catheterization, or coronary angiography.

Your doctor will give you specific instructions about how to prepare for surgery. He or she will advise you about what to eat or drink, what medicines to take, and what activities to stop (such as smoking). You'll likely be admitted to the hospital on the day of the surgery.

If tests for coronary heart disease show you have severe blockages in your coronary (heart) arteries, your doctor may admit you to the hospital right away. You may have CABG that day or the day after.

What to Expect during Coronary Artery Bypass Grafting

CABG requires a team of experts. A cardiothoracic surgeon does the surgery with support from an anesthesiologist, a perfusionist (heart-lung bypass machine specialist), other surgeons, and nurses.

There are several types of CABG. They range from traditional surgery, in which the chest is opened to reach the heart, to nontraditional surgery in which small incisions are made to bypass the blocked or narrowed artery.

Traditional CABG

This type of surgery usually lasts three to five hours, depending on the number of arteries being bypassed. Numerous steps take place during traditional CABG.

You'll be under general anesthesia for the surgery. The term *anesthesia* refers to a loss of feeling and awareness. General anesthesia temporarily puts you to sleep.

During the surgery, the anesthesiologist checks your heartbeat, blood pressure, oxygen levels, and breathing. A breathing tube is placed in your lungs through your throat. The tube is connected to a ventilator (a machine that helps you breathe).

An incision is made down the center of your chest. The chest bone is then cut and your rib cage is opened so the surgeon can get to your heart. Medicine is used to stop your heart, which allows the surgeon to operate on it while it's not beating. You're also given medicine to protect your heart function during the time it's not beating. A heart-lung bypass machine keeps oxygen-rich blood moving throughout your body during the surgery.

An artery or vein is taken from your body—for example, from your chest or leg—and is prepared as a graft for the bypass. In surgery with several bypasses, both artery and vein grafts are commonly used.

Artery grafts are much less likely than vein grafts to become blocked over time. The left internal mammary artery most often is used for an artery graft. It's located inside the chest, close to the heart. Arteries from the arm or other places in the body are sometimes used as well.

Although veins are also commonly used as grafts, they're more likely than artery grafts to develop plaque and become blocked over time. The saphenous vein—a long vein running along the inner side of the leg—is typically used.

After the grafting procedure, blood flow to your heart is restored. Usually the heart starts beating again on its own. In some cases, mild electric shocks are used to restart the heart. You're then disconnected from the heart-lung bypass machine. Tubes are inserted into your chest to drain fluid.

The surgeon uses wires to close your chest bone (much like how a broken bone is repaired). The wires stay in your body permanently. After your chest bone heals, it will be as strong as it was before the surgery.

Stitches or staples are used to close the skin incision. The breathing tube is removed when you're able to breathe without it.

Nontraditional CABG

Nontraditional CABG includes off-pump CABG and minimally invasive CABG. Off-pump CABG, which does not stop the heart and does not use a heart-lung bypass machine, can be used to bypass any of the coronary arteries. When off-pump CABG is used, the part of the heart where grafting is being done is steadied with a mechanical device.

There are several types of minimally invasive direct coronary artery bypass (MIDCAB) grafting. These types of surgery differ from traditional bypass surgery. They require only small incisions rather than opening the chest bone to get to the heart. These procedures sometimes use a heart-lung bypass machine. The different types of MIDCAB grafting are as follows:

- **MIDCAB procedure:** This procedure is used when only one or two coronary arteries need to be bypassed. A series of small incisions is made between your ribs on the left side of your chest, directly over the artery to be bypassed. The incisions usually are about 3 inches long. (The incision made in traditional CABG is at least 6 to 8 inches long.) The left internal mammary artery most often is used for the graft. A heart-lung bypass machine isn't used during this procedure.

- **Port-access coronary artery bypass procedure:** This procedure is done through small incisions (ports) made in your chest. Artery or vein grafts are used. A heart-lung bypass machine is used during this procedure.

- **Robot-assisted technique:** This type of procedure allows for even smaller, keyhole-sized incisions. A small video camera is inserted in one incision to show the heart, while the surgeon uses remote-controlled surgical instruments to do the surgery. A heart-lung bypass machine is sometimes used during this procedure.

Nontraditional CABG procedures have been developed to improve upon problems associated with traditional methods. They appear to speed recovery, but studies have not clearly showed better overall results.

What to Expect after Coronary Artery Bypass Grafting

Recovery in the Hospital

After surgery, you'll typically spend one or two days in an ICU. Your heart rate, blood pressure, and oxygen levels will be checked regularly during this time.

An IV line will likely be inserted into a vein in your arm. Through the IV line, you may get medicines to control blood circulation and blood pressure. You also will likely have a tube in your bladder to drain urine and a tube to drain fluid from your chest.

You may receive oxygen therapy (oxygen given through nasal prongs or a mask) and a temporary pacemaker while in the ICU. A pacemaker is a small device that's placed in the chest or abdomen to help control abnormal heart rhythms.

Your doctor may recommend that you wear compression stockings on your legs as well. These stockings are tight at the ankle and become looser as they go up the leg, which creates gentle pressure up the leg. The pressure keeps blood from pooling and clotting.

While in the ICU, you'll also have bandages on your chest incision and on the areas where an artery or vein was removed for grafting. After you leave the ICU, you'll be moved to a less intensive care area of the hospital for three to five days before going home.

Recovery at Home

Your doctor will give you specific instructions for recovering at home, especially concerning how to care for your healing incisions, how to recognize signs of infection or other complications, when to call the doctor right away, and when to make follow-up appointments.

You also may get instructions on how to deal with common side effects of surgery. Side effects often go away within four to six weeks after surgery but may include discomfort or itching from healing incisions, swelling of the area where an artery or vein was removed for grafting, muscle pain or tightness in the shoulders and upper back, and fatigue, mood swings, or depression. Some people also experience problems sleeping or loss of appetite, constipation, and chest pain around the site of the chest bone incision (more frequent with traditional CABG). Full recovery from traditional CABG may take 6 to 12 weeks or more. Less recovery time is needed for nontraditional CABG.

Your doctor will tell you when you can start physical activity again. It varies from person to person, but there are some typical time frames. Most people can resume sexual activity within about four weeks and driving after three to eight weeks.

Returning to work after six weeks is common unless your job involves specific and demanding physical activity. Some people may need to find less physically demanding types of work or work a reduced schedule at first.

Ongoing Care

Care after surgery may include periodic checkups with doctors. During these visits, tests may be done to see how your heart is working. Tests may include an EKG, stress testing, echocardiography, and cardiac computed tomography (CT).

CABG is not a cure for CHD. You and your doctor may develop a treatment plan that includes lifestyle changes to help you stay healthy and reduce the chance of your CHD getting worse. Lifestyle changes may include making changes to your diet, quitting smoking, doing physical activity regularly, and lowering and managing stress. These strategies are discussed in chapters 29–36.

Your doctor also may refer you to cardiac rehabilitation (rehab). Cardiac rehab is a medically supervised program that helps improve the health and well-being of people who have heart problems. Rehab programs include exercise training, education on heart-healthy living, and counseling to reduce stress and help you return to an active life. Doctors supervise these programs, which may be offered in hospitals and other community facilities. Talk to your doctor about whether cardiac rehab might benefit you. Chapter 28 has more information on cardiac rehab.

Taking medicine as prescribed also is an important part of care after surgery. Your doctor may prescribe medicines to manage pain during recovery, lower cholesterol and blood pressure, reduce the risk of blood clots forming, manage diabetes, or treat depression.

Risks of Coronary Artery Bypass Grafting

Although complications from CABG are uncommon, the risks include wound infection and bleeding, reactions to anesthesia, fever, pain, and stroke, heart attack, or even death.

Some patients develop a fever associated with chest pain, irritability, and decreased appetite. This is due to inflammation involving the lungs and heart sac. This complication sometimes is seen one to six weeks after surgeries that involve cutting through the pericardium (the outer covering of the heart). This reaction usually is mild. However, some patients may develop fluid buildup around the heart that requires treatment.

Memory loss and other changes, such as problems concentrating or thinking clearly, may occur in some people. These changes are more likely to occur in people who are older, who have high blood pressure or lung disease, or who drink excessive amounts of alcohol. These side effects often improve several months after surgery.

The use of a heart-lung bypass machine increases the risk of blood clots forming in your blood vessels. Clots can travel to the brain or other parts of the body and block the flow of blood, which may cause a stroke or other problems. Recent technical improvements in heart-lung bypass machines are helping reduce the risk of blood clots.

In general, the risk of complications is higher if CABG is done in an emergency situation (for example, during a heart attack), if you're older than 70, or if you have a history of smoking. Your risk also is higher if you have other diseases or conditions, such as diabetes, kidney disease, lung disease, or peripheral arterial disease.

Adapted from "Coronary Artery Bypass Grafting," National Heart, Lung, and Blood Institute (NHLBI, www.nhlbi.nih.gov), January 2010.

Implantable Defibrillators

An implantable cardioverter defibrillator (ICD) is a small device that's placed in your chest or abdomen. The device uses electrical pulses or shocks to help control life-threatening, irregular heartbeats, especially those that could cause sudden cardiac arrest (SCA).

SCA is a condition in which the heart suddenly and unexpectedly stops beating. If the heart stops beating, blood stops flowing to the brain and other vital organs, which usually causes death if it's not treated in minutes.

ICDs use electrical pulses or shocks to treat life-threatening arrhythmias that occur in the ventricles (the heart's lower chambers). When ventricular arrhythmias occur, the heart can't effectively pump blood. You can pass out within seconds and die within minutes if not treated. To prevent death, the condition must be treated right away with an electric shock to the heart. This treatment is called defibrillation.

Doctors also treat arrhythmias with another type of device called a pacemaker. An ICD is similar to a pacemaker, but there are some differences. Pacemakers can give off only low-energy electrical pulses. They're often used to treat less dangerous heart rhythms, such as those that occur in the upper chambers of your heart (for more information about pacemakers, see chapter 25). Most new ICDs can act as both pacemakers and defibrillators.

Patients who have heart failure may need a special device called a cardiac resynchronization therapy (CRT) device. The CRT device is able to pace both ventricles at the same time. This allows them to work together and do a better job pumping blood out of the heart. CRT devices that have a defibrillator are called CRT-D.

When an Implantable Cardioverter Defibrillator Is Necessary

ICDs are used to treat life-threatening ventricular arrhythmias, such as those that cause the ventricles to beat too fast or quiver. You may be considered at high risk for a ventricular arrhythmia if you have had a ventricular arrhythmia before or you have had a heart attack that has damaged your heart's electrical system.

ICDs often are recommended for people who have survived SCA. People who have certain heart conditions that put them at high risk for SCA also may need ICDs. For example, some people who have long QT syndrome, Brugada syndrome, or congenital heart disease may benefit from an ICD, even if they've never had ventricular arrhythmias.

How an Implantable Cardioverter Defibrillator Works

An ICD has wires with electrodes on the ends that connect to one or more of your heart's chambers. These wires carry the electrical signals from your heart to a computer in the ICD that monitors your heart rhythm.

If the ICD detects an irregular rhythm, it sends low-energy electrical pulses to prompt your heart to beat at a normal rate. If the low-energy pulses restore your heart's normal rhythm, you may avoid the high-energy pulses or shocks of the defibrillator (which can be painful).

Single-chamber ICDs have a wire that connects to either the right atrium or right ventricle. The wire senses electrical activity and corrects faulty electrical signaling within that chamber.

Dual-chamber ICDs have wires that connect to both an atrium and a ventricle. These ICDs provide low-energy pulses to either or both chambers. Some dual-chamber ICDs have three wires. They connect to an atrium and both ventricles.

The wires on an ICD connect to a small metal box implanted in your chest or abdomen. The box contains a battery, a pulse generator, and a computer. When the computer detects irregular heartbeats, it triggers the ICD's pulse generator to send electrical pulses. Wires carry these pulses to the heart.

The ICD also can record the heart's electrical activity and heart rhythms. The recordings can help your doctor fine-tune the programming of your ICD so it works better to correct irregular heartbeats.

The type of ICD you get is based on your heart's pumping abilities, structural defects, and the type of irregular heartbeats you've had. Whichever type of ICD you get, it will be programmed to respond to the type of irregular heartbeat you're most likely to have.

What to Expect during Implantable Cardioverter Defibrillator Surgery

Placing an ICD requires minor surgery, which usually is done in a hospital. You'll be given medicine right before the surgery that will help you relax and may make you fall asleep.

Your doctor will give you medicine to numb the area where he or she will put the ICD so you don't feel any pain. Your doctor also may give you antibiotics to prevent infection.

First, your doctor will thread the ICD wires through a vein to the correct location in your heart. An x-ray movie of the wires as they pass through your vein and into your heart will help your doctor place them.

Once the wires are in place, your doctor will make a small cut into the skin of your chest or abdomen. He or she will then slip the ICD's small metal box through the cut and just under your skin. The box contains the battery, the pulse generator, and the computer.

Once the ICD is in place, your doctor will test it. You'll be given medicine to help you sleep during this testing so you won't feel any electrical pulses. Then your doctor will sew up the cut. The entire surgery takes a few hours.

What to Expect after Implantable Cardioverter Defibrillator Surgery

Expect to stay in the hospital one to two days so your health care team can check your heartbeat and make sure your ICD is working properly.

You'll need to arrange for a ride home from the hospital because you won't be able to drive for at least a week while you recover from the surgery.

For a few days to weeks after the surgery, you may have pain, swelling, or tenderness in the area where your ICD was placed. The pain usually is mild, and over-the-counter medicines can help relieve it. Talk to your doctor before taking any pain medicine.

Your doctor may ask you to avoid vigorous activities and heavy lifting for about a month after ICD surgery. Most people return to their normal activities within a few days of having the surgery.

Risks of Having an Implantable Cardioverter Defibrillator

Unnecessary Electrical Pulses

The most common problem with ICDs is that they can sometimes give electrical pulses or shocks that aren't needed.

A damaged wire or a very fast heart rate due to extreme physical activity may trigger unnecessary pulses. Unnecessary pulses also may occur if you forget to take your medicine.

Children tend to be more physically active than adults, and younger people who have ICDs are more likely to receive unnecessary pulses than older people.

Pulses delivered too often or at the wrong time can damage the heart or trigger an irregular, sometimes dangerous heartbeat. They also can be painful and emotionally upsetting. If this occurs, your doctor can reprogram your ICD or prescribe medicine so the unnecessary pulses occur less often.

Risks Related to Surgery

Although rare, some ICD risks are linked to the surgery used to place the device. These risks include swelling, bruising, or infection at the area where the ICD was placed; bleeding from the site where the ICD was placed; blood vessel, heart, or nerve damage; a collapsed lung; and a negative reaction to the medicine used to make you sleep during the surgery.

Other Risks

People who have ICDs may be at increased risk for heart failure. Heart failure is when your heart can't pump enough blood to meet your body's needs. It's not known for sure whether an ICD increases the risk of heart failure or whether heart failure is just more common in people who need ICDs.

Although rare, an ICD may not work properly, which could prevent the device from correcting irregular heartbeats. If this happens, your doctor may be able to reprogram the device. If that doesn't work, the ICD may need to be replaced.

The longer you have an ICD, the more likely you'll experience some of the related risks.

Living with an Implantable Cardioverter Defibrillator

The low-energy electrical pulses your ICD gives aren't painful. You may not notice them, or you may feel a fluttering in your chest.

The high-energy pulses or shocks your ICD gives last only a fraction of a second and feel like a thumping or painful kick in the chest, depending on their strength.

Your doctor may give you medicine to decrease the number of irregular heartbeats you have. This will reduce the number of high-energy pulses sent to your heart. Such medicines include amiodarone or sotalol and beta blockers.

Your doctor may want you to call his or her office or come in within 24 hours of getting a strong shock from your ICD. See your doctor or go to an emergency room right away if you get many strong shocks within a short time.

Devices That Can Disrupt Implantable Cardioverter Defibrillator Functions

Once you have an ICD, you have to avoid close or prolonged contact with electrical devices or devices that have strong magnetic fields. Devices that can interfere with an ICD include cell phones and MP3 players (for example, iPods), some household appliances such as microwave ovens, high-tension wires, metal detectors, industrial welders, and electrical generators. These devices can disrupt the electrical signaling of your ICD and prevent it from working properly. You may not be able to tell whether your ICD has been affected.

How likely a device is to disrupt your ICD depends on how long you're exposed to it and how close it is to your ICD. To be on the safe side, some experts recommend not putting your cell phone or MP3 player (if it's turned on) in a shirt pocket over your ICD. You may want to hold your cell phone up to the ear opposite the site where your ICD was implanted. If you strap your MP3 player to your arm while listening to it, put it on the arm farther from your ICD.

You can still use household appliances, but avoid close and prolonged exposure, as it may interfere with your ICD.

You can walk through security system metal detectors at your normal pace. Someone can check you with a metal detector wand as long as it isn't held for too long over your ICD site. You should avoid sitting or standing close to a security system metal detector. Notify airport screeners if you have an ICD.

Stay at least two feet away from industrial welders or electrical generators. Rarely, ICDs have caused inappropriate shocks during long, high-altitude flights.

Procedures That Can Disrupt Implantable Cardioverter Defibrillator Functions

Some medical procedures can disrupt your ICD. These procedures include magnetic resonance imaging (MRI), shock-wave lithotripsy to treat kidney stones, and electrocauterization to stop bleeding during surgery.

Let all your doctors, dentists, and medical technicians know you have an ICD. Your doctor can give you a card that states what kind of ICD you have. Carry this card in your wallet. You may want to consider wearing a medical ID bracelet or necklace that explains you have an ICD.

Maintaining Daily Activities

Physical Activity

In most cases, having an ICD won't limit you from taking part in sports and exercise, including strenuous activities. You may need to avoid full-contact sports, such as football. Such contact could damage your ICD or shake loose the wires in your heart. Ask your doctor how much and what kinds of physical activity are safe for you.

Driving

You'll be asked to avoid driving for at least a week while you recover from ICD surgery. If you've had sudden cardiac arrest, a ventricular arrhythmia, or certain symptoms of a ventricular arrhythmia (such as fainting), your doctor may ask you not to drive until you have gone six months without fainting. Some people may still faint even with an ICD. Commercial driving isn't permitted with an ICD.

Ongoing Care

Your doctor will want to check your ICD regularly. Over time, your ICD may stop working properly if its wires get dislodged or broken, its battery fails, your heart disease progresses, or other devices have disrupted its electrical signaling.

To check your ICD, your doctor may ask you to come in for an office visit several times a year. Some ICD functions can be checked remotely through a telephone call or a computer connection to the internet.

Your doctor also may recommend an EKG to check for changes in your heart's electrical activity.

Battery Replacement

ICD batteries last between five and seven years. Your doctor will replace the generator along with the battery before the battery begins to run down. Replacing the generator/battery is a less involved surgery than the original surgery to implant the ICD. The wires of your ICD also may need to be replaced eventually. Your doctor can tell you whether you need to replace your ICD or its wires.

Benefits of Having an Implantable Cardioverter Defibrillator

An ICD is very effective at detecting and stopping certain life-threatening arrhythmias. An ICD can work better than drug therapy at preventing sudden cardiac arrest, depending on the cause of the arrest.

Although an ICD can't cure heart disease, it can lower the risk of dying by up to 50% in some patients who have heart disease.

Adapted from "Implantable Cardioverter Defibrillator," National Heart, Lung, and Blood Institute (NHLBI, www.nhlbi.nih.gov), August 2009.

Chapter 25

Pacemakers

A pacemaker is a small device placed in the chest or abdomen to help control abnormal heart rhythms. This device uses electrical pulses to prompt the heart to beat at a normal rate.

Pacemakers are used to treat arrhythmias. For more information about arrhythmias, see chapter 4. A pacemaker can relieve some arrhythmia symptoms, such as fatigue and fainting. A pacemaker also can help a person who has abnormal heart rhythms resume a more active lifestyle.

Understanding Pacemakers

Faulty electrical signaling in the heart causes arrhythmias. A pacemaker uses low-energy electrical pulses to overcome this faulty electrical signaling. Pacemakers can do the following things:

- Speed up a slow heart rhythm
- Help control an abnormal or fast heart rhythm

- Make sure the ventricles contract normally if the atria are quivering instead of beating with a normal rhythm (a condition called atrial fibrillation)

- Coordinate the electrical signaling between the upper and lower chambers of the heart

- Coordinate the electrical signaling between the ventricles; pacemakers that do this are called cardiac resynchronization therapy (CRT) devices and are used to treat heart failure

- Prevent dangerous arrhythmias caused by a disorder called long QT syndrome

Pacemakers also can monitor and record your heart's electrical activity and heart rhythm. Newer pacemakers can monitor your blood temperature, breathing rate, and other factors and adjust your heart rate to changes in your activity.

Pacemakers can be temporary or permanent. Temporary pacemakers are used to treat temporary heartbeat problems, such as a slow heartbeat caused by a heart attack, heart surgery, or an overdose of medicine.

Temporary pacemakers also are used during emergencies. They're used until a permanent pacemaker can be implanted or until the temporary condition goes away. If you have a temporary pacemaker, you'll stay in a hospital as long as the device is in place.

Permanent pacemakers are used to control long-term heart rhythm problems. Except where noted, this chapter discusses permanent pacemakers.

Doctors also treat arrhythmias with other devices called implantable cardioverter defibrillators (ICDs). An ICD is similar to a pacemaker. However, besides using low-energy electrical pulses, an ICD also can use high-energy electrical pulses to treat certain dangerous arrhythmias. For more information about ICDs, see chapter 24.

When a Pacemaker Is Necessary

Doctors recommend pacemakers for a number of reasons. The most common reasons are bradycardia and heart block. Bradycardia is a slower than normal heartbeat. Heart block is a problem with the heart's electrical system that occurs when an electrical signal is slowed or disrupted as it moves through the heart.

Your doctor also may recommend a pacemaker if any of the following are true:

- Aging or heart disease has damaged your sinus node's ability to set the correct pace for your heartbeat. Such damage can cause slower than normal heartbeats or long pauses between heartbeats. The damage also can cause your heart to alternate between slow and fast rhythms. This condition is called sick sinus syndrome.

- You've had a medical procedure to treat an arrhythmia called atrial fibrillation. A pacemaker can help regulate your heartbeat after the procedure.

- You need to take certain heart medicines, such as beta blockers. These medicines may slow your heartbeat too much.

- You faint or have other symptoms of a slow heartbeat. For example, this may happen if the main artery in your neck that supplies your brain with blood is sensitive to pressure. Just quickly turning your neck can cause your heart to beat slower than normal. If this happens, not enough blood may flow to your brain, causing you to feel faint or collapse.

- You have heart muscle problems that cause electrical signals to travel too slowly through your heart muscle. (Your pacemaker may provide cardiac resynchronization therapy for this problem.)

- You have long QT syndrome, which puts you at risk for dangerous arrhythmias.

Children, adolescents, and people who have certain types of congenital heart disease may get pacemakers. Pacemakers also are sometimes implanted after heart transplants.

Before recommending a pacemaker, your doctor will consider any arrhythmia symptoms you have, such as dizziness, unexplained fainting, or shortness of breath. He or she also will consider whether you have a history of heart disease, what medicines you're currently taking, and the results of heart tests.

How a Pacemaker Works

A pacemaker system consists of a battery, a computerized generator, and wires with sensors called electrodes on one end. The battery powers the generator, and both are surrounded by a thin metal box. The wires connect the generator to the heart.

A pacemaker monitors and helps control your heartbeat. The electrodes detect your heart's electrical activity and send data through the wires to the computer in the generator.

If your heart rhythm is abnormal, the computer will direct the generator to send electrical pulses to your heart. The pulses then travel through the wires to reach your heart. Newer pacemakers also can monitor your blood temperature, breathing, and other factors and adjust your heart rate to changes in your activity.

The pacemaker's computer also records your heart's electrical activity and heart rhythm. Your doctor will use these recordings to adjust your pacemaker so it works better for you. Your doctor can program the pacemaker's computer with an external device. He or she doesn't have to use needles or have direct contact with the pacemaker.

Pacemakers have one to three wires that are each placed in different chambers of the heart. The wires in a single-chamber pacemaker usually carry pulses between the right ventricle (the lower right chamber of your heart) and the generator.

The wires in a dual-chamber pacemaker carry pulses between the right atrium (the upper right chamber of your heart) and the right ventricle and the generator. The pulses help coordinate the timing of these two chambers' contractions.

The wires in a biventricular pacemaker carry pulses between an atrium and both ventricles and the generator. The pulses help coordinate electrical signaling between the two ventricles. This type of pacemaker also is called a cardiac resynchronization therapy device.

The two main types of programming for pacemakers are demand pacing and rate-responsive pacing. A demand pacemaker monitors your heart rhythm. It sends electrical pulses to your heart only if your heart is beating too slow or if it misses a beat. A rate-responsive pacemaker will speed up or slow down your heart rate depending on how active you are. To do this, the rate-responsive pacemaker monitors your sinus node rate, breathing, blood temperature, and other factors to determine your activity level.

Most people who need pacemakers to continually set the pace of their heartbeats have rate-responsive pacemakers.

What to Expect during Pacemaker Surgery

Placing a pacemaker requires minor surgery. The surgery usually is done in a hospital or special heart-treatment laboratory. Before the surgery, an IV line will be inserted into one of your veins. Medicine will be given through the IV line to help you relax. The medicine also may make you sleepy.

Your doctor will give you medicine to numb the area where he or she will put the pacemaker so you don't feel any pain. Your doctor also may give you antibiotics to prevent infection.

First, your doctor will place a needle in a large vein, usually near the shoulder opposite your dominant hand. Your doctor will then use the needle to thread the pacemaker wires into the vein and to the correct place in your heart.

An x-ray movie of the wires as they pass through your vein and into your heart will help your doctor place them correctly. Once the wires are in place, your doctor will make a small cut into the skin of your chest or abdomen.

He or she will then slip the pacemaker's small metal box through the cut, place it just under your skin, and connect it to the wires that lead to your heart. The box contains the pacemaker's battery and generator.

Once the pacemaker is in place, your doctor will test it to make sure it works properly. He or she will then sew up the cut. The entire surgery takes a few hours.

What to Expect after Pacemaker Surgery

Expect to stay in the hospital overnight so your health care team can check your heartbeat and make sure your pacemaker is working properly. You'll probably have to arrange for a ride to and from the hospital because your doctor may not want you to drive yourself.

For a few days to weeks after surgery, you may have pain, swelling, or tenderness in the area where your pacemaker was placed. The pain usually is mild, and over-the-counter medicines often relieve it. Talk to your doctor before taking any pain medicine.

Your doctor may ask you to avoid vigorous activities and heavy lifting for about a month after pacemaker surgery. Most people return to their normal activities within a few days of the surgery.

Risks of Pacemaker Surgery

Your chance of having any problems from pacemaker surgery is very low. If problems do occur, they may include swelling, bleeding, bruising, or infection in the area where the pacemaker was placed; blood vessel or nerve damage; a collapsed lung; or a negative reaction to the medicine used during the procedure.

Living with a Pacemaker

Once you have a pacemaker, you have to avoid close or prolonged contact with electrical devices or devices that have strong magnetic fields. Devices that can interfere with a pacemaker include cell phones and MP3 players (for example, iPods), household appliances such as microwave ovens, high-tension wires, metal detectors, industrial welders, and electrical generators.

These devices can disrupt the electrical signaling of your pacemaker and stop it from working properly. You may not be able to tell whether your pacemaker has been affected. How likely a device is to disrupt your pacemaker depends on how long you're exposed to it and how close it is to your pacemaker.

To be on the safe side, some experts recommend not putting your cell phone or MP3 player (if it's turned on) in a shirt pocket over your pacemaker. You may want to hold your cell phone up to the ear opposite the site where your pacemaker was implanted. If you strap your MP3 player to your arm while listening to it, put it on the arm farther from your pacemaker.

You can still use household appliances, but avoid close and prolonged exposure, as it may interfere with your pacemaker.

You can walk through security system metal detectors at your normal pace. You also can be checked with a metal detector wand as long as it isn't held for too long over your pacemaker site. You should avoid sitting or standing close to a security system metal detector. Notify airport screeners if you have a pacemaker.

Stay at least 2 feet away from industrial welders or electrical generators.

Some medical procedures can disrupt your pacemaker. These procedures include magnetic resonance imaging (MRI), shock-wave lithotripsy to get rid of kidney stones, and electrocauterization to stop bleeding during surgery.

Let all your doctors, dentists, and medical technicians know you have a pacemaker. Your doctor can give you a card that states what kind of pacemaker you have. Carry this card in your wallet. You may want to consider wearing a medical ID bracelet or necklace that states you have a pacemaker.

Physical Activity

In most cases, having a pacemaker won't limit you from doing sports and exercise, including strenuous activities. You may need to avoid full-contact sports, such as football. Such contact could damage your pacemaker or shake loose the wires in your heart. Ask your doctor how much and what kinds of physical activity are safe for you.

Ongoing Care

Your doctor will want to check your pacemaker regularly (about every three months). Over time, a pacemaker can stop working properly if its wires get dislodged or broken, its battery gets weak or fails, your heart disease progresses, or other devices have disrupted its electrical signaling.

To check your pacemaker, your doctor may ask you to come in for an office visit several times a year. Some pacemaker functions can be checked remotely through a telephone call or a computer connection to the Internet.

Your doctor also may ask you to have an EKG to check for changes in your heart's electrical activity.

Battery Replacement

Pacemaker batteries last between 5 and 15 years (average 6 to 7 years), depending on how active the pacemaker is. Your doctor will replace the generator along with the battery before the battery starts to run down.

Replacing the generator/battery is a less involved surgery than the original surgery to implant the pacemaker. The wires of your pacemaker also may need to be replaced eventually. Your doctor can tell you whether your pacemaker or its wires need to be replaced when you see him or her for follow-up visits.

Adapted from "Pacemaker," National Heart, Lung, and Blood Institute (NHLBI, www.nhlbi.nih.gov), December 2009.

Chapter 26

Heart Transplant

A heart transplant is surgery to remove a person's diseased heart and replace it with a healthy heart from a deceased donor. Ninety percent of heart transplants are done on patients who have end-stage heart failure. For more information about heart failure, see chapter 3.

The Heart Transplant Process

The heart transplant process starts when doctors refer patients to a heart transplant center for evaluation. Patients found to be eligible for a heart transplant are placed on a waiting list for a donor heart.

Heart transplant surgery is done in a hospital when a suitable donor heart is found. After the transplant, patients are started on a lifelong health care plan. The plan involves multiple medicines and frequent medical checkups.

When a Heart Transplant Is Necessary

Referral to a Heart Transplant Center

Most patients referred to a heart transplant center have end-stage heart failure. Of these patients, close to half have heart failure as a result of coronary heart disease. Others have heart failure caused by hereditary conditions, viral infections of the heart, or damaged heart valves and muscles. (Some medicines, alcohol, and pregnancy can damage the heart valves and muscles.)

Most patients considered for a heart transplant have tried other, less drastic treatments and have been hospitalized a number of times for heart failure.

Eligibility for Heart Transplant

The heart transplant specialists at the heart transplant center will determine whether a patient is eligible for a transplant. Specialist teams often include a cardiologist (a doctor who specializes in diagnosing and treating heart problems), a cardiovascular surgeon (a doctor who does the transplant surgery), a transplant coordinator (a person who makes arrangements for the surgery, such as transportation of the donor heart), a social worker, a dietitian, and a psychiatrist.

In general, patients selected for heart transplants have severe end-stage heart failure but are healthy enough to have the transplant. Heart failure is considered end stage when all possible treatments—such as medicine, implanted devices, and surgery—have failed.

Patients who have the following conditions might not be candidates for heart transplant surgery because the procedure is less likely to be successful:

- Advanced age (although there's no widely accepted upper age limit for a heart transplant, most transplant surgery is done on patients younger than 70 years old)
- Poor blood circulation throughout the body, including the brain

- Kidney, lung, or liver diseases that can't be reversed
- History of cancer or malignant tumors
- Inability or unwillingness to follow lifelong medical instructions after a transplant
- Pulmonary hypertension (high blood pressure in the lungs) that can't be reversed
- Active infection throughout the body

What to Expect before a Heart Transplant

The Heart Transplant Waiting List

Patients who are eligible for a heart transplant are placed on a waiting list for a donor heart. This waiting list is part of a national allocation system for donor organs run by the Organ Procurement and Transplantation Network (OPTN).

OPTN has policies in place to make sure donor hearts are given out fairly. These policies are based on urgency of need, the organs available for transplant, and the location of the patient receiving the heart (the recipient). Organs are matched for blood type and size of donor and recipient.

The Donor Heart

Guidelines on how a donor heart is selected require that the donor meet the legal requirement for brain death and that the appropriate consent forms are signed.

Guidelines suggest that the donor be younger than 65 years old, have little or no history of heart disease or trauma to the chest, and not be exposed to hepatitis or HIV. The guidelines also recommend that the donor heart not be without blood circulation for more than four hours.

Waiting Times

Approximately 3,000 people in the United States are on the waiting list for a heart transplant on any given day. About 2,000 donor hearts are available each year. Wait times vary from days to several months and will depend on a recipient's blood type and condition.

A person may be taken off the list for some time if he or she has a serious medical event such as a stroke, infection, or kidney failure.

Time spent on the waiting list plays a part in who receives a donor heart. For example, if a donor heart becomes available and two recipients have equal need, the recipient who has been waiting longer usually will get the heart.

Ongoing Medical Treatment

Patients on the waiting list for a donor heart receive ongoing treatment for heart failure and other medical conditions. Treating arrhythmias (irregular heartbeats), for example, is very important because they can cause sudden cardiac arrest in people who have heart failure.

As a result, many transplant centers will place implantable cardioverter defibrillators (ICDs) in patients before surgery. An ICD is a small device that's placed in the chest or abdomen to help control life-threatening arrhythmias.

Another treatment that may be recommended to waiting-list patients is an implanted mechanical pump called a ventricular assist device (VAD). This device helps the heart pump blood.

Regular outpatient care for waiting-list patients may include frequent exercise testing, assessing the strength of the heartbeat, and right cardiac catheterization (a test to measure blood pressure in the right side of the heart).

Contact with the Transplant Center during the Wait

People on the waiting list often are in close contact with their transplant centers. Most donor hearts must be transplanted within four hours after removal from the donor.

At some heart transplant centers, recipients get a pager so the center can contact them at any time. They're asked to tell the transplant center staff if they're going out of town. Recipients often need to be prepared to arrive at the hospital within two hours of being notified about a donor heart.

Not all patients who are called to the hospital will get a heart transplant. Sometimes, at the last minute, doctors find that a donor heart isn't suitable for a patient. Other times, patients from the waiting list are called to come in as possible substitutes in case something happens with the selected recipient.

What to Expect during a Heart Transplant

Just before the heart transplant surgery, patients will get general anesthesia. General anesthesia temporarily puts you to sleep.

A bypass machine is hooked up to the arteries and veins of the heart. The machine pumps blood through the patient's lungs and body while the diseased heart is removed and the donor heart is sewn into place.

Heart transplant surgery usually takes about four hours. Patients often spend the first days after surgery in the intensive care unit of the hospital.

What to Expect after a Heart Transplant

In the Hospital

The amount of time a heart transplant recipient spends in the hospital will vary with each person. It often involves one to two weeks in the hospital and three months of monitoring by the transplant team at the heart transplant center.

Monitoring may include frequent blood tests, lung function tests, EKGs, echocardiograms, and biopsies of the heart tissue.

A heart biopsy is a standard test used to see whether your body is rejecting the new heart. It might be done often in the weeks after a transplant.

During a heart biopsy, a tiny grabbing device is inserted into a vein in the neck or groin (upper thigh). The device is threaded through the vein to the right atrium of the new heart to take a small tissue sample. The tissue sample is checked for signs of rejection.

While in the hospital, your health care team may recommend that you start a cardiac rehabilitation (rehab) program. Cardiac rehab is a medically supervised program that helps improve the health and well-being of people who have heart problems. Cardiac rehab includes counseling, education, and exercise training to help you recover. Rehab may start with a member of the rehab team helping you sit up in a chair or take a few steps. Over time, you'll increase your activity level.

Watching for Signs of Rejection

The new heart is a foreign body that your immune system may attack if you're not getting enough medicine to suppress your immune system after the surgery. You and the transplant team will work together to protect the new heart by watching for signs of rejection. These signs include shortness of breath, fever, fatigue, weight gain (retaining fluid in the body), and reduced amounts of urine (caused by problems in the kidneys).

You and the team also will work together to manage the transplant medicines and their side effects, prevent infections, and continue treatment of ongoing medical conditions. You may be asked to check your temperature, blood pressure, and pulse when you go home.

Preventing Rejection

You'll need to take medicine to suppress your immune system so it doesn't reject the new heart. These transplant medicines are called immunosuppressants. They're a combination of medicines tailored to your situation. Often they include cyclosporine, tacrolimus, mycophenolate mofetil (MMF), and steroids such as prednisone. Your doctors may need to change or adjust your transplant medicines if they aren't working well or if you have too many side effects.

Managing Transplant Medicines and Their Side Effects

You'll have to manage multiple medicines. It's helpful to set up a routine for taking medicines at the same time each day and for refilling prescriptions. It's crucial to never run out of medicine. Always using the same pharmacy may help.

Keep a list of all your medicines with you at all times in case of an accident. When traveling, keep extra doses of medicine with you, not packed in your luggage. Bring your medicines with you to all doctor visits.

Side effects from medicine can be serious. Side effects include risk of infection, diabetes, osteoporosis (thinning of the bones), high blood pressure, kidney disease, and cancer—especially lymphoma and skin cancer.

Discuss any side effects of your medicines with your transplant team. Your doctors may change or adjust your medicines if you're having problems. Make sure your doctors know all the medicines you're taking.

Preventing Infection

Some transplant medicines can increase your risk of infection. You may be asked to watch for signs of infection, including fever, sore throat, cold sores, and flu-like symptoms. Signs of possible chest or lung infections could include shortness of breath, cough, and a change in the color of your sputum (spit).

The incision from your surgery must be checked for redness, swelling, or drainage. It's especially important to look for signs of infection because transplant medicines often mask these signs.

Talk to your doctor about what steps you should take to reduce your risk of infection. For example, your doctor may recommend that you avoid contact with animals or crowds of people in the first few months after your transplant.

Regular dental care also is important. Your doctor may prescribe antibiotics before any dental work to prevent infections.

Pregnancy

Many successful pregnancies have occurred after heart transplant surgeries; however, special care is important. If you've had a heart transplant, talk with your doctor before planning a pregnancy.

Emotional Issues and Support

Having a heart transplant may cause fear, anxiety, and stress. While you're waiting for a heart transplant, you may worry you won't live long enough to get a new heart. After surgery, you may feel overwhelmed, depressed, or worried about complications.

All these feelings are normal for someone going through major heart surgery. It's important to talk about how you feel with your health care team. Talking to a professional counselor also can help. If you're feeling very depressed, your health care team or counselor may prescribe medicines to make you feel better.

Support from family and friends also can help relieve stress and anxiety. Let your loved ones know how you feel and what they can do to help you.

Risks of Heart Transplant

Although heart transplant surgery is a life-saving measure, it has many risks. Careful monitoring, treatment, and regular medical care can prevent or help manage some of these risks.

Failure of the Donor Heart

Over time, the new heart may fail due to the same factors that caused the original heart to fail. Failure of the donor heart also can occur if your body rejects the donor heart or if cardiac allograft vasculopathy, described later in this section, develops.

Patients who have a heart transplant that fails can be considered for another transplant (called a retransplant).

Primary Graft Dysfunction

The most frequent cause of death in the first 30 days after transplant is primary graft dysfunction. This occurs if the new donor heart fails and isn't able to function.

Factors such as shock or trauma to the donor heart or narrowed blood vessels in the recipient's lungs can cause primary graft dysfunction. Medicines (for example, inhaled nitric oxide and intravenous nitrates) may be used to treat this condition.

Rejection of the Donor Heart

Rejection is one of the leading causes of death in the first year after transplant. The recipient's immune system sees the new heart as a foreign body and attacks it.

During the first year, 25% of heart transplant patients have signs of a possible rejection at least once. Half of all possible rejections happen in the first six weeks after surgery, and most happen within six months of surgery.

Cardiac Allograft Vasculopathy

Cardiac allograft vasculopathy (CAV) is a chronic disease in which the walls of the coronary arteries in the new heart become thick, hard, and lose their elasticity. CAV can destroy blood circulation in the new heart and cause serious damage.

CAV is a leading cause of donor heart failure and death in the years following transplant surgery. CAV can cause heart attack, heart failure, dangerous arrhythmias, and sudden cardiac arrest.

To detect CAV, your doctor may recommend coronary angiography yearly as well as other tests, such as stress echocardiography or intravascular ultrasound.

Complications from Medicines

Taking daily medicines that stop the immune system from attacking the new heart is absolutely critical even though the medicine combinations have serious side effects.

Cyclosporine and other medicines can cause kidney damage. Kidney damage affects more than 25% of patients in the first year after transplant. Five percent of transplant patients will develop end-stage kidney disease within seven years.

Infection

When the immune system—the body's defense system—is suppressed, the risk of infection increases. Infection is a major cause of hospital admission for heart transplant patients and a leading cause of death in the first year after transplant.

Cancer

Suppressing the immune system leaves patients at risk for cancers and malignancies. Malignancies are a major cause of late death in heart transplant patients, accounting for nearly 25% of heart transplant deaths three years after transplant.

The most common malignancies are tumors of the skin and lips (patients at highest risk are older, male, and fair skinned) and malignancies in the lymph system, such as non-Hodgkin lymphoma.

Other Complications

High blood pressure develops in more than 70% of heart transplant patients in the first year after transplant and in nearly 95% of patients within five years.

High levels of cholesterol and triglycerides in the blood develop in more than 50% of heart transplant patients in the first year after transplant and in 84% of patients within five years.

Osteoporosis can develop or worsen in heart transplant patients. This condition thins and weakens the bones.

Complications from Not Following a Lifelong Health Care Plan

Not following a lifelong health care plan increases the risk of all heart transplant complications. Heart transplant patients are asked to closely follow their doctors' instructions and check their own health status throughout their lives.

Lifelong health care includes taking multiple medicines on a strict schedule, watching for signs and symptoms of complications, keeping all medical appointments, and stopping unhealthy behaviors (such as smoking).

Adapted from "Heart Transplant," National Heart, Lung, and Blood Institute (NHLBI, www.nhlbi.nih.gov), October 2009.

Part Three

Moving Forward

Finding out you have heart disease can be a life-changing event, but the changes need not be limiting. In fact, with appropriate care and attention to certain issues, the changes you make can help you achieve levels of health and fitness that surpass what you experienced before your diagnosis. This part of the book looks to the future and discusses what may await you.

If you have suffered a heart attack or undergone heart surgery, you will want to know what to expect during your recovery and rehabilitation. The opening chapter in this part explains your first weeks at home after you've been hospitalized for care. It describes the practical and emotional challenges you may encounter as you begin to resume your usual activities. The next chapter describes the process of cardiac rehabilitation, the people who may be on your rehab team, and how they can help you reach your long-term health-related goals.

For most people with heart disease, an important part of the recovery process involves addressing lifestyle issues. The next chapters provide positive, proactive steps for taking better care of your heart. Here you'll find detailed discussions about the importance of physical activity, healthy eating, and controlling medical conditions that could harm your heart, especially high blood pressure, high cholesterol, and diabetes. And if your recovery efforts are being thwarted because of struggles with weight management, smoking cessation, or stress, you will find chapters that offer encouragement and tips for overcoming these challenges.

In addition to lifestyle issues, you may have ongoing health care needs that require additional care. Angina and sexual dysfunction are two of particular importance because of their widespread occurrence. A chapter on angina offers details about identifying its triggers and making appropriate activity adjustments. It also discusses the medications and additional medical procedures that may be needed. A chapter on managing sexual problems discusses how doctors evaluate and treat the most common difficulties.

Finally, one of the most important steps in living with heart disease is developing an action plan for dealing with potential future emergencies. This part concludes with a chapter about heart attack warning signs and the need to plan ahead for seeking immediate medical help. It also reviews facts about cardiopulmonary resuscitation (CPR), offers tips for finding CPR classes, and discusses automated external defibrillators.

Chapter 27

Your Recovery after a Heart Attack or Heart Procedure

Having a heart attack or a heart procedure can be a frightening and upsetting experience. It is difficult to discover—often suddenly—that your body isn't working the way it should and to be plunged into an unfamiliar world of hospitals and high-tech procedures. But it's important to know that millions of people have survived heart problems, recovered fully, and gone on to resume active, normal lives.

Likewise, most people who undergo heart surgery recover well and return to their usual activities. Many surgery patients eventually feel healthier than they did before their procedures.

The time it takes to get back to normal will depend on many factors, including your age and general health. If you have had a heart attack, your pace of recovery will also depend on the severity of the attack, and if you have undergone surgery, your recovery time will depend partly on the type of procedure you had.

But whatever your situation, there is much you can do to improve your health and prevent complications following a heart attack or major heart procedure.

The first step: give yourself permission to recover. You and your body have been through a lot, and it will take some time to feel like yourself again. Expect to feel quite tired at first and to gradually regain your strength and energy. While individual needs vary, following are some overall tips for successful recovery after a heart attack or heart surgery.

Your First Weeks at Home

When you first arrive home from the hospital, you'll need to get a lot of rest so your heart can begin to heal. It is very important to eat healthy foods and get enough sleep. Take the medications your doctor has prescribed for you. Avoid heavy yard work, house cleaning, or other projects that require a lot of energy. Also refrain from physical activity in very hot or cold weather. Ask family and friends to help out with chores, child care, and other activities that may be difficult to take care of during your first weeks at home.

At the same time, it is important to get up and move around as you begin to recover. Your heart is a muscle that needs to be exercised—though very gently at first. Pace yourself. Allow plenty of time for each thing you do during the day, from getting out of bed to taking a shower to preparing a simple breakfast. Rest between activities and whenever you feel tired. Ask your doctor for a list of guidelines for activity during your first few weeks at home.

Your doctor will want to check your progress one to four weeks after you leave the hospital. During your first follow-up visit, your doctor will check your weight and blood pressure, make any needed changes in your medicines, perform necessary tests, and check the overall progress of your recovery. Use this opportunity to ask any questions you may have about safe or unsafe activities, medicines, lifestyle changes, or any other issues that concern you. You may want to write down your questions beforehand.

For some situations and questions, it is best to call your doctor right away rather than wait for your next appointment. Call promptly if you experience the following:

- You have symptoms related to your original heart disease, such as trouble breathing, chest pain, weakness, or an irregular heartbeat.

- You notice side effects after starting a new heart medicine.

- You've been given a prescription for a condition other than heart disease. It is important to find out whether it's safe to take other medicines along with your heart drugs.

- You've recently had heart surgery or another kind of medical treatment and you notice symptoms your doctor has warned you about.

- You feel down or have the blues for more than a few days.

If you have symptoms of a possible heart attack, call 911 right away.

Getting Your Life Back

As you begin to recover from a heart attack or heart procedure, you may naturally wonder when you can return to your usual activities, including work, sexual activity, driving, and travel. Most people can safely return to most of their normal activities within a few weeks as long as they do not have chest pain or other complications.

While you should ask your doctor when you can return to each of your usual activities, here are some general guidelines.

Work

Most people are able to return to their usual work within several weeks. Your doctor may ask you to take tests to find out if you can do the kind of job you did before. While most individuals can continue their customary work with no problems, some people choose to change jobs or reduce their hours to lighten the load on their heart. Counselors at cardiac rehab programs may be able to provide support and resources for those considering a job change.

Sexual Activity

Most people can resume sexual relations about three to six weeks after a heart attack or heart procedure as long they have no chest pain or other complications. But since everyone recovers at his or her own pace, your doctor may give you a stress test to determine when you can safely resume sexual activity. When you're ready for sex again, choose a time when you feel relaxed and rested. Wait at least an hour after eating a full meal to allow time for digestion.

Take your time. If you have chest pain or other heart symptoms during sexual activity, have lost interest, or are worried about having sex, talk with your doctor.

A special note: Couples who use medication to enhance sex should know that these drugs can cause irregular heartbeats. If you've been using one of these medicines or are considering taking one, ask your doctor whether it is safe to do so.

Driving

Driving can usually begin within a week for most patients, if allowed by state law. Each state has its own regulations for driving a motor vehicle following a serious illness, so contact your state's Department of Motor Vehicles for guidelines. People with complications or chest pain should not drive until their symptoms have been stable for a few weeks.

Travel

Once your doctor tells you it's safe for you to travel, keep these tips in mind:

- Keep your medications in your purse or carry-on luggage so they will be easily available when you need them.

- Pack light so you can lift your luggage without strain. At the airport, train, or bus station, use a pull-cart to cut down on lifting. If possible, get help from a porter.

- Allow more time than usual to catch your flight, train, or bus.

- Walk around at least every two hours during trips. While sitting, flex your feet frequently and do other simple exercises to increase blood flow in your legs and prevent blood clots.

- Check with your doctor before traveling to locations at high altitudes (greater than 6,000 feet) or places where the temperature will be either very hot or very cold. When you first arrive, give yourself a chance to rest.

Remember, each person's recovery process is different. Don't try to guess when you can return to normal activities. Always ask your doctor first.

Coping with Your Feelings

Anyone who has had a heart attack or has undergone heart surgery knows it can be an upsetting experience. You've just come through a major health crisis, and your usual life has been disrupted.

Afterward, it's normal to experience a wide range of feelings. You may feel some relief. But you may also feel worried, angry, or depressed. It may be reassuring to know that these reactions are very common and that most difficult feelings pass within a few weeks. Here are some things to remember:

- Take one day at a time. Try not to think too much about next week or next month. Do what you can do today. Enjoy small pleasures: a walk in your neighborhood, a conversation with a loved one, a snuggle with a pet, or a good meal.

- Share your concerns. Talk with family members and friends about your feelings and concerns, and ask for support. Be sure to ask for the kind of support you need. (For example, if you want a sympathetic ear rather than advice, gently let your loved ones know.)

- Be sure to give family members time to say what they feel and need, too. Supportive relationships may actually help lengthen life after a heart attack.

- Get support from veterans. Whether you've had a heart attack or gone through heart surgery, consider joining a support group for people who have shared your experience. Groups for heart patients can provide emotional support as well as help you develop new ways of handling everyday challenges. For a list of support groups in your local area, contact Mended Hearts at www.mendedhearts. org or at 888-432-7899. Your local American Heart Association chapter may also offer support groups.

- Keep moving. Regular physical activity not only helps reduce the risk of future heart problems but also helps relieve anxiety, depression, and other difficult feelings. Any regular physical activity—even gentle walking—can help lift your mood.

- Seek help for depression. Up to 20% of heart disease patients battle serious depression, and many more suffer milder cases of the blues. If you find yourself feeling very sad or discouraged for more than a week or so, be sure to let your doctor know. Counseling and/or medication can often be very helpful. Seeking help is very important, not only because you deserve to enjoy life as fully as possible, but also because heart patients who are successfully treated for depression are less likely to have future serious heart problems.

Reviewed for currency and excerpted from "Your Guide to Living Well with Heart Disease," National Heart, Lung, and Blood Institute (NHLBI, www.nhlbi .nih.gov), November 2005.

Chapter 28

Cardiac Rehabilitation

Cardiac rehabilitation (rehab) is a medically supervised program that helps improve the health and well-being of people who have heart problems. Rehab programs include exercise training, education on heart-healthy living, and counseling to reduce stress and help you return to an active life.

Cardiac rehab helps people who have heart problems in the following ways:

- It helps them recover after a heart attack or heart surgery.

- It helps them prevent future hospital stays, heart problems, and death related to heart problems.

- It helps them address risk factors that lead to coronary heart disease (also called coronary artery disease) and other heart problems. These risk factors include high blood pressure, high blood cholesterol, overweight or obesity, diabetes, smoking, lack of physical activity, and depression and other emotional health concerns.

- It helps them adopt healthy lifestyle changes. These changes may include a heart-healthy diet, increased physical activity, and stress management.

- It helps them improve their health and quality of life.

Each patient will have a program that's designed to meet his or her needs.

The Team

Cardiac rehab involves a long-term commitment from the patient and a team of health care providers.

The cardiac rehab team may include doctors (such as a family doctor, a heart specialist, and a surgeon), nurses, exercise specialists, physical and occupational therapists, dietitians or nutritionists, and psychologists or other mental health specialists. In some cases, a case manager will help track the patient's care.

Working with the team is an important part of cardiac rehab. The patient should share questions and concerns with the team, which will help the patient reach his or her goals.

When It's Needed

People of all ages and ethnic backgrounds can benefit from cardiac rehab. The lifestyle changes made during rehab have few risks. These changes can improve your overall health and prevent future heart problems and even death.

Exercise training as part of cardiac rehab may not be safe for all patients. For example, people who have very high blood pressure or severe heart disease may not be ready to exercise. These patients can still benefit from other parts of the cardiac rehab program.

Ask your doctor whether cardiac rehab can help you prevent a future heart problem and improve your health. Rehab may help people who have had a heart attack, angioplasty or coronary artery bypass grafting for coronary heart disease, heart valve repair or replacement, a heart or lung transplant, stable angina, or heart failure.

Cardiac rehab is equally helpful for both men and women. It can improve your overall health and prevent future heart problems and even death.

What to Expect

Your doctor may refer you to cardiac rehab during an office visit or while you're in the hospital recovering from a heart attack or heart surgery. If your doctor doesn't mention it, ask him or her whether cardiac rehab might benefit you.

Rehab activities vary depending on your condition. If you're recovering from major heart surgery, rehab will start with a member of the rehab team helping you sit up in a chair or take a few steps. You'll work on range-of-motion exercises. These include moving your fingers, hands, arms, legs, and feet. Over time, you'll increase your activity level.

Once you leave the hospital, rehab will continue in a rehab center. The rehab center may be part of the hospital or in another place.

Try to find a center close to home that offers services at a convenient time. If no centers are near your home, or if it's too hard to get to them, ask your doctor about home-based rehab.

For the first two to three months, you'll need to go to rehab regularly to learn how to reduce risk factors and begin an exercise program. After that, your rehab team may recommend less frequent visits.

Overall, you may work with the rehab team for 12 months or more. The length of time you continue cardiac rehab depends on your situation.

Health Assessment

Before you start your cardiac rehab program, your rehab team will assess your health. This includes taking your medical history and doing a physical exam and tests.

A doctor or nurse will ask you about previous heart problems, heart surgery, and any heart-related symptoms you have. He or she also will ask whether you've had medical procedures or other health problems (such as diabetes or kidney disease).

The doctor or nurse may ask whether your family has a history of heart disease; what medicines you're taking, including over-the-counter medicines and dietary supplements (such as vitamins and herbal remedies); and how much, how often, and when you take each medicine. You may also be asked whether you smoke and how much. If you have diabetes, you may be asked how you check your blood sugar level, how often you do it, and whether you've ever had hypoglycemia (low blood sugar levels that can occur in people who take medicine to control their blood sugar).

Your rehab team will also ask questions to help them assess your quality of life and well-being.

A doctor or nurse will do a physical exam to check your overall health, including your heart rate, blood pressure, reflexes, and breathing.

Your doctor may recommend tests to check your heart. A resting EKG is a simple test that detects and records your heart's electrical activity. It shows how fast your heart is beating, your heart's rhythm (steady or irregular), and the strength and timing of electrical signals as they pass through each part of your heart. You also may need tests to measure your cholesterol and blood sugar levels. If you have diabetes, staff also will do an HbA1C test to check your blood sugar control. This test shows how well your diabetes has been managed over time.

Lifestyle Changes

During cardiac rehabilitation, you'll learn how to increase your physical activity and exercise safely, follow a heart-healthy diet, reduce risk factors for future heart problems, and improve your emotional health. The rehab team will work with you to create a plan that meets your needs. Each part of cardiac rehab will help lower your risk for future heart problems.

Over time, the lifestyle changes you make during rehab will become more routine. They will help you maintain a reduced risk for heart disease.

Support from your family can help make cardiac rehab easier. For example, family members can help you plan healthy meals and do physical activities. The healthy lifestyle changes you learn during cardiac rehab can benefit your entire family.

Physical Activity and Exercise

Physical activity is an important part of a healthy lifestyle. It can strengthen your heart muscle, reduce your risk for heart disease, and improve your muscle strength, flexibility, and endurance.

Your rehab team will assess your physical activity level to learn how active you are at home, at work, and during recreation. If your job includes heavy labor, the team may re-create your workplace conditions to help you practice in a safe setting.

You'll work with the team to find ways to safely add physical activity to your daily routine. For example, you may decide to park farther from building entrances, walk up two or more flights of stairs, or walk for 15 minutes during your lunch break.

Your rehab team also will work with you to create an easy-to-follow exercise plan. It will include time for a warm-up, flexibility exercises, and cooling down. It also may include aerobic exercise and muscle-strengthening activities. You'll get a written plan that lists each exercise and explains how often and for how long you should do it.

You're more likely to make exercise a habit if you enjoy the activity. Work with the rehab team to find the types of activity that you enjoy and that are safe for you. If you prefer to exercise with other people, join a group or ask a friend to join you.

Exercise training as part of cardiac rehab may not be safe for all patients. For example, if you have very high blood pressure or severe heart disease, you may not be ready for exercise training. Or you may only be able to tolerate very light conditioning exercises. The rehab team will help decide what level of exercise is safe for you.

Aerobic Exercise

Typically, your rehab team will ask you to do aerobic exercise three to five days per week for 30 to 60 minutes. The exercise specialist on your team will make sure your exercise plan is safe and right for you. Examples of aerobic exercise are walking (outside or on a treadmill), cycling, rowing, or climbing stairs.

Muscle-Strengthening Activities

Typically, your rehab team will ask you to do muscle-strengthening activities two or three days per week. Your exercise plan will show how many times to repeat each exercise. Muscle-strengthening activities may include lifting weights (hand weights, free weights, or weight machines), using a wall pulley, or using elastic bands to stretch and condition your muscles.

Exercise at the Rehab Center and at Home

When you start cardiac rehab, you'll exercise at the rehab center. Members of your rehab team will carefully watch you to make sure you're exercising safely.

A team member will check your blood pressure several times during exercise training. You also may need an EKG to check your heart's electrical activity during exercise. This test shows how fast your heart is beating and whether its rhythm is steady or irregular.

Your exercise program will change as your health improves. After awhile, you'll add at-home exercises to your plan. You can find more information about physical activity and heart health in chapter 29.

Diet

Your rehab team will help you create and follow a heart-healthy diet. The diet will help you reach your rehab goals, which may include managing your weight, cholesterol levels, blood pressure, diabetes, kidney disease, heart failure, and/or other health problems your diet can affect. You'll learn how to plan meals that meet your calorie needs and are low in saturated and trans fats, cholesterol, and sodium (salt). Chapter 30 offers additional information about heart-healthy eating.

Your rehab team also may advise you to limit alcohol and other substances. Alcohol can raise your blood pressure and harm your liver, brain, and heart.

Reduce Risk Factors

Your cardiac rehab team will work with you to control your risk factors for heart problems. Risk factors include high blood pressure, high blood cholesterol, overweight or obesity, diabetes, and smoking.

Improve Emotional Health

Psychological factors increase the risk of getting heart disease or making it worse. Depression, anxiety, and anger are common among people who have heart disease or have had a heart attack or heart surgery.

Get treatment if you feel sad, anxious, angry, or isolated. These feelings can affect your physical recovery. Depression is linked to complications such as irregular heartbeats, chest pain, a longer recovery time, the need to return to the hospital, and even an increased risk of death.

Seeking help is important. Group or individual counseling helps lower your risk for future heart attacks and death. It also may motivate you to exercise and help you relax and learn how to reduce stress.

People with heart disease who get mental health treatment often show improvements in blood pressure, cholesterol, and other measures of physical health.

The rehab team may include a mental health specialist, or someone from the team may be able to refer you to one. Without help from a professional, these problems may not go away.

Some communities have support groups for people who have had heart attacks or heart surgery. They also may have walking groups or exercise classes. Help with basic needs and transportation also may be available.

Risks of Cardiac Rehabilitation

The lifestyle changes you make during cardiac rehab have few risks. At first, physical activity is safer in the rehab setting than at home. Members of the rehab team are trained and have experience teaching people who have heart problems how to exercise.

Your rehab team will watch you to make sure you're safe. They'll check your blood pressure several times during your exercise training. They also may use an EKG to see how your heart reacts and adapts to exercise. After some training, most people learn to exercise safely at home.

Very rarely, physical activity during rehab causes serious problems. These problems may include injuries to your muscles and/or bones or heart rhythm problems that can lead to death or recurrent heart attack.

Your rehab team will tell you about signs and symptoms to watch for while exercising at home. If you notice these signs and symptoms, you should stop the activity and contact your doctor.

Reviewed for currency and excerpted from "Cardiac Rehabilitation," National Heart, Lung, and Blood Institute (NHLBI, www.nhlbi.nih.gov), August 2009.

Chapter 29

Physical Activity and Your Heart

Physical activity is any body movement that works your muscles and uses more energy than you use when resting. Walking, running, dancing, swimming, yoga, and gardening are examples of physical activity.

According to the Department of Health and Human Services' "2008 Physical Activity Guidelines for Americans," physical activity generally refers to bodily movement that enhances health.

Exercise is a type of physical activity that's planned and structured. Lifting weights, taking an aerobics class, and playing on a sports team are examples of exercise.

Physical activity is good for many parts of your body. Being physically active, along with following a healthy diet and not smoking, are the most important things you can do to keep your heart and lungs healthy.

Many Americans are not active enough. The good news, though, is that even modest amounts of physical activity are good for your health. The more active you are, the more you will benefit.

Types of Physical Activity

The four main types of physical activity are aerobic, muscle strengthening, bone strengthening, and stretching. Aerobic activity is the type that benefits your heart and lungs the most.

Aerobic Activity

Aerobic activity moves your large muscles, such as those in your arms and legs. Running, swimming, walking, bicycling, dancing, and doing jumping jacks are examples of aerobic activity. Aerobic activity also is called endurance activity.

Aerobic activity makes your heart beat faster than usual. You also breathe harder during this type of activity. Over time, regular aerobic activity makes your heart and lungs stronger and able to work better.

Other Types of Physical Activity

The other types of physical activity—muscle strengthening, bone strengthening, and stretching—benefit your body in other ways.

Muscle-strengthening activities improve the strength, power, and endurance of your muscles. Doing push-ups and sit-ups, lifting weights, climbing stairs, and digging in the garden are examples of muscle-strengthening activities.

With bone-strengthening activities, your feet, legs, or arms support your body's weight, and your muscles push against your bones. This helps make your bones strong. Running, walking, jumping rope, and lifting weights are examples of bone-strengthening activities.

Muscle-strengthening and bone-strengthening activities also can be aerobic, depending on whether they make your heart and lungs work harder than usual. For example, running is both an aerobic activity and a bone-strengthening activity.

Stretching helps improve your flexibility and your ability to fully move your joints. Touching your toes, doing side stretches, and doing yoga exercises are examples of stretching.

Levels of Intensity

You can do aerobic activity with light, moderate, or vigorous intensity. In healthy people, moderate- and vigorous-intensity aerobic activities are better for your heart than light-intensity activities. However, even light-intensity activities are better than no activity at all.

The level of intensity depends on how hard you have to work to do the activity. To do the same activity, people who are less fit usually have to work harder than people who are more fit. So, for example, what is light-intensity activity for one person may be moderate-intensity for another.

Light-intensity activities are common daily activities that don't require much effort. Moderate-intensity activities make your heart, lungs, and muscles work harder than light-intensity activities do.

On a scale of 0 to 10, moderate-intensity activity is a 5 or 6 and produces noticeable increases in breathing and heart rate. A person doing moderate-intensity activity can talk but not sing.

Vigorous-intensity activities make your heart, lungs, and muscles work hard. On a scale of 0 to 10, vigorous-intensity activity is a 7 or 8. A person doing vigorous-intensity activity can't say more than a few words without stopping for a breath.

Examples of Aerobic Activities

Examples of aerobic activities include pushing a grocery cart around a store, gardening that causes your heart rate to go up (such as digging or hoeing), walking, hiking, jogging, running, water aerobics, swimming laps, bicycling, skateboarding, rollerblading, jumping rope, ballroom dancing, aerobic dancing, tennis, soccer, hockey, and basketball. Depending on your level of fitness, they can be light, moderate, or vigorous in intensity.

Benefits

Physical activity, especially aerobic activity, is good for your heart and lungs in many ways. The benefits of physical activity apply to people of all ages and races and both sexes.

Moderate- and vigorous-intensity physical activity done regularly strengthens your heart muscle. This improves your heart muscle's ability to pump blood to your lungs and throughout your body. As a result, more blood flows to your muscles, and oxygen levels in your blood rise.

Capillaries, your body's tiny blood vessels, also widen. This allows them to deliver more oxygen to your body and carry away waste products, such as carbon dioxide and lactic acid.

Moderate- and vigorous-intensity aerobic activity done regularly can lower your risk for coronary heart disease (CHD). Certain traits, conditions, or habits may raise your risk for CHD. Physical activity can help control some of these risk factors because it does the following:

- It can lower blood pressure.

- It helps improve and manage levels of cholesterol and other fats in the blood. Physical activity can lower triglyceride levels. Triglycerides are a type of fat. Physical activity also can raise high-density lipoprotein (HDL), or good, cholesterol levels.

- It improves your body's ability to manage blood sugar and insulin levels. This lowers your risk for type 2 diabetes.

- It reduces levels of C-reactive protein (CRP) in your body. This protein is a sign of inflammation. High levels of CRP may raise your risk for CHD.

- It helps reduce overweight and obesity when combined with reduced calorie intake. Physical activity also helps you maintain a healthy weight over time.

- It may help people quit smoking. Smoking is a major risk factor for CHD.

Inactive people are nearly twice as likely to develop CHD as people who are physically active. Studies suggest that like high blood cholesterol, high blood pressure, and smoking, inactivity is a major risk factor for CHD.

In people who have CHD, regular aerobic activity helps the heart work better. It also may reduce the risk of a second heart attack in people who already have had a heart attack.

Vigorous aerobic activity may not be safe for people who have CHD. Talk to your doctor about what type of activity is safe for you.

Risks

In general, the benefits of regular physical activity far outweigh risks to the heart and lungs.

Rarely, heart problems—such as arrhythmia, sudden cardiac arrest, or heart attack—occur during physical activity. These events generally happen to people who already have heart conditions.

For youth and young adults, the risk for heart problems due to physical activity is higher in people who have underlying congenital heart problems—heart problems present since birth.

Congenital heart problems include hypertrophic cardiomyopathy, congenital heart defects, and myocarditis. People who have these conditions should talk to their doctors about which physical activities are safe for them.

In middle-aged and older adults, the risk for heart problems due to physical activity is related to coronary heart disease. People who already have CHD are more likely to have a heart attack when they're exercising vigorously than when they're not.

The risk for heart problems due to physical activity is related to your fitness level and the intensity of the activity you're doing. For example, someone who doesn't do physical activity regularly is at higher risk for heart attack during vigorous activity than a person who is physically fit and regularly active.

If you have a heart problem or chronic disease, such as heart disease, diabetes, or high blood pressure, talk to your doctor about what types of physical activity are safe for you. You also should talk to your doctor about safe physical activities if you have symptoms such as chest pain or dizziness. Discuss ways to slowly and safely build physical activity into your daily routine.

Getting Started and Staying Active

Physical activity is an important part of a heart-healthy lifestyle, but talk to your doctor before you get started if you have heart disease or another chronic health condition.

Do It Daily

You don't have to become a marathon runner to get all the benefits of physical activity. Do activities you enjoy, and make them part of your daily routine.

If you haven't been active for a while, start low and build slow. Many people like to start with walking and slowly increase their time and distance. You also can take other steps to make physical activity part of your routine.

You can make your daily routine more active. For example, take the stairs instead of the elevator. Instead of sending e-mails, walk down the hall to a co-worker's office. Rake the leaves instead of using a leaf blower.

Identify Benefits

People value different things. Some people may highly value the health benefits of physical activity. Others want to be active because they enjoy recreational activities or want to look or sleep better.

Some people want to be active because it helps them lose weight or gives them a chance to spend time with friends. Identify which physical activity benefits you value. This will help you personalize the benefits of physical activity.

Involve Friends and Family

Friends and family can help you stay active. For example, go for a hike with a friend. Take dancing lessons with your spouse, or play ball with your child. The possibilities are endless.

Reward Yourself

Sometimes going for a bike ride or a long walk relieves stress after a long day. Think of physical activity as a special time to refresh your body and mind.

Consider keeping a log of your activity. A log can help you track your progress. Many people like to wear a pedometer (a small device that counts steps) to track how much they walk every day. These tools can help you set goals and stay motivated.

Be Safe

Physical activity is safe for almost everyone. You can take steps to make sure it's safe for you too.

- Be active on a regular basis to raise your fitness level.

- Do activities that fit your health goals and fitness level. Start low and slowly increase your activity level over time. As your fitness improves, you will be able to do physical activities for longer periods and with more intensity.

- Spread out your activity over the week and vary the types of activity you do.

- Use the right gear and equipment to protect yourself. For example, use bicycle helmets, elbow and knee pads, and goggles.

- Be active in safe environments. Pick well-lit and well-maintained places clearly separated from car traffic.

- Follow safety rules and policies, such as always wearing a helmet when biking.

- Make sensible choices about when, where, and how to be active. Consider weather conditions, such as how hot or cold it is, and change your plans as needed.

Talk to Your Doctor

If you have a heart problem or chronic disease, such as heart disease, diabetes, or high blood pressure, talk to your doctor about what types of physical activity are safe for you.

You also should talk to your doctor about safe physical activities if you have symptoms such as chest pain or dizziness.

Reviewed for currency and excerpted from "Physical Activity and Your Heart," National Heart, Lung, and Blood Institute (NHLBI, www.nhlbi.nih.gov), May 2009.

Chapter 30

Heart-Healthy Eating

What you eat affects your risk for heart disease and poor blood circulation, which can lead to a heart attack.

Foods You Should Eat

You should eat mainly the following types of foods:

- Fruits and vegetables

- Grains (at least half of your grains should be whole grains, such as whole wheat, whole oats, oatmeal, whole-grain corn, brown rice, wild rice, whole rye, whole-grain barley, buckwheat, bulgur, millet, quinoa, and sorghum)

- Fat-free or low-fat varieties of milk, cheese, yogurt, and other milk products

- Fish, skinless poultry, lean meats, dry beans, eggs, and nuts

- Polyunsaturated and monounsaturated fats (found in fish, nuts, and vegetable oils)

Also, you should limit the amount of foods you eat that contain the following:

- Saturated fat (found in foods such as fatty cuts of meat, whole milk, cheese made from whole milk, ice cream, sherbet, frozen yogurt, butter, lard, cakes, cookies, doughnuts, sausage, regular mayonnaise, coconut, and palm oil)

- Trans fat (found mainly in processed foods such as cakes, cookies, crackers, pies, stick or hard margarine, potato chips, and corn chips)

- Cholesterol (found in foods such as liver, chicken and turkey giblets, pork, sausage, whole milk, cheese made from whole milk, ice cream, sherbet, and frozen yogurt)

- Sodium (found in salt and baking soda)

- Added sugars (such as corn syrup, corn sweetener, fructose, glucose, sucrose, dextrose, lactose, maltose, honey, molasses, raw sugar, invert sugar, malt syrup, syrup, caramel, and fruit juice concentrates)

A diet high in saturated fat, trans fat, and cholesterol may cause plaque buildup in your arteries. Eating lots of sodium may cause you to develop high blood pressure, also called hypertension. Too many added sugars may cause you to develop type 2 diabetes. Both hypertension and diabetes increase your risk of heart disease and stroke.

Prepared foods that come in packages—such as breads, cereals, canned and frozen foods, snacks, desserts, and drinks—have Nutrition Facts labels. These labels state how many calories and how much saturated fat, trans fat, and other substances are in each serving.

For food that does not have a Nutrition Facts label, such as fresh salmon or a raw apple, you can use the U.S. Department of Agriculture (USDA) National Nutrient Database (www.nal.usda.gov/fnic/foodcomp/search). This is a bit harder than using the Nutrition

Facts label. But by comparing different foods you can get an idea if a food is high or low in saturated fat, sodium, and other substances.

Calories

A calorie of food is a measure of the energy the food supplies to your body. When talking about burning calories during physical activity, a calorie is a measure of the energy used by your body. To maintain the same body weight, the number of food calories you eat during the day should be about the same as the number of calories your body uses.

The number of calories you should eat each day depends on your age, sex, body size, level of physical activity, and other conditions. For instance, a woman between the ages of 31 and 50 who is of normal weight and moderately active should eat about 2,000 calories each day. For additional information about daily calorie intake, see chapter 34.

Eating Plans

There are four eating plans that can help you choose heart-healthy foods: MyPyramid eating plan, Dietary Approaches to Stop Hypertension (DASH) eating plan, Heart-Healthy Diet, and Therapeutic Lifestyle Changes (TLC) Diet.

The MyPyramid eating plan is based on the Dietary Guidelines for Americans. It was developed by the USDA and the U.S. Department of Health and Human Services to help people lower their risk of serious diseases linked to diet, including heart disease. DASH was developed by the National Heart, Lung, and Blood Institute (NHLBI) to help people with hypertension lower their blood pressure. But it can also be used to help prevent heart disease. The Heart-Healthy Diet was developed by NHLBI to help people keep their blood levels of total cholesterol and LDL cholesterol (low-density lipoprotein, or bad, cholesterol) low. The TLC diet was

developed by NHLBI to help people with unhealthy blood cholesterol levels.

The four eating plans are similar. They are all designed to help you
eat foods that are good for your heart and avoid foods that are bad
for your heart. Table 30.1 compares the main guidelines of the four
eating plans.

Heart-Healthy Eating Plans

More information on these eating plans, including interactive tools to
help you choose foods that meet their guidelines, is available online:

- www.mypyramid.gov
- www.nhlbi.nih.gov

Sodium

All four eating plans limit the amount of sodium you should eat
each day. Populations who consume diets low in salt do not experience the increase in blood pressure with age seen in most Western
countries.

Sodium chloride is the chemical name for salt. The words *salt* and
sodium are not exactly the same, yet these words are often used in
place of each other. For example, the Nutrition Facts panel uses
sodium, whereas the front of a package may say *low salt*.

Ninety percent of the sodium we consume is in the form of salt.

Sodium Consumption and Sodium in Our Food Supply

We all need a small amount (for example, 180 mg per day) of sodium to keep our bodies working properly.

The 2005 Dietary Guidelines for Americans recommend limiting
sodium to less than 2,300 mg per day (about 1 tsp of table salt). The

Table 30.1. Heart-Healthy Eating Plans: How They Compare

	% of the day's total calories from saturated fat	% of the day's total calories from fat	amount of trans fat	milligrams (mg) of dietary cholesterol per day	milligrams (mg) of dietary sodium per day
MyPyramid	less than 10%	20–35%	as low as possible	less than 300 mg	less than 2,300 mg*
DASH**	5%	22%	as low as possible	136 mg	less than 2,300 mg*
Heart-Healthy Diet	8–10%	30% or less	as low as possible	less than 300 mg	less than 2,400 mg
TLC Diet	less than 7%	25–35% or less	as low as possible	less than 200 mg	less than 2,400 mg

*2,300 mg of sodium in table salt is about 1 tsp of salt. People with hypertension should eat no more than 1,500 mg of sodium a day (about 2/3 tsp of salt). African Americans and middle-aged and older adults should also eat no more than 1,500 mg of sodium per day because these groups have a high risk of developing hypertension.

**These DASH guidelines are for someone eating 2,000 calories each day.

guidelines further recommend that specific populations (African Americans, persons with high blood pressure, and middle-aged and older adults) consume no more than 1,500 mg per day (about 2/3 tsp of table salt). These specific populations account for about 70% of adults.

The average daily sodium intake for Americans age two years and older is 3,436 mg.

The majority of the sodium consumed is from processed and restaurant foods; only a small portion is used in cooking or added at the table.

Sodium content can vary significantly within food categories. For example, a regular slice of frozen cheese pizza can range from 450 mg to 1,200 mg, and some brands of breakfast sausage links have twice the sodium content of other brands.

Nutrition labeling and packaging messages are easily misunderstood by consumers. Sodium information is not readily available for restaurant foods and can be hard for consumers to estimate. For example, consumers might be surprised to find the restaurant salad they are consuming may contain more than 900 mg of sodium—and they might only be able to find this information on the company's website.

Reducing Sodium

Make sure to check the sodium content on the Nutrition Facts label when buying food. Choosing the brands with lower sodium content can be one way to lower the amount of sodium you eat.

Another way to limit sodium is to use spices other than salt. There are plenty of salt-free spice combinations in your grocery store. It may take a while for you to get used to the taste, but give it time. After a while, you may like them better than salt.

Besides limiting the amount of sodium you eat, it is also a good idea to eat foods rich in potassium. A potassium-rich diet blunts the harmful effects of sodium on blood pressure. Aim to eat 4,700 mg of potassium a day. Foods rich in potassium include fruits and vegetables, especially tomatoes and tomato products; orange juice and grapefruit juice; raisins; dates; prunes; white potatoes; sweet potatoes; lettuce; and papayas.

Omega-3 Fatty Acids

Fish and shellfish contain a type of fat called omega-3 fatty acids. Research suggests eating omega-3 fatty acids lowers your chances of dying from heart disease. Fish that naturally contain more oil (such as salmon, trout, herring, mackerel, anchovies, and sardines) have more omega-3 fatty acids than lean fish (such as cod, haddock, and catfish). Be careful, though, about eating too much shellfish. Shrimp, for example, is a type of shellfish that has a lot of cholesterol.

You can also get omega-3 fatty acids from plant sources, such as canola oil, soybean oil, walnuts, and ground flaxseed (linseed) and flaxseed oil.

Alcohol

Drinking too much alcohol can, over time, damage your heart and raise your blood pressure. If you drink alcohol, you should do so moderately. For women, moderate drinking means one drink per day. For men, it means two drinks per day. One drink counts as the following:

- 5 ounces of wine
- 12 ounces of beer
- 1.5 ounces of 80-proof hard liquor

Research suggests moderate drinkers are less likely to develop heart disease than people who don't drink any alcohol or who drink too much. Red wine drinkers in particular seem to be protected to some degree against heart disease. Red wine contains flavonoids, which are thought to prevent plaque buildup. Flavonoids also are found in red grapes, berries, apples, and broccoli.

On the other hand, drinking more than one drink per day increases the risks of certain cancers, including breast cancer. And if you are pregnant, could become pregnant, or have another health condition that could make alcohol use harmful, you should not drink.

With the help of your doctor, decide whether moderate drinking to lower heart attack risk outweighs the possible increased risk of breast cancer or other medical problems.

Getting Help

If you need help working out an eating plan that's right for you, you may want to talk with a registered dietitian. A dietitian is a nutrition expert who can give you advice about what foods to eat and how much of each type. Ask your doctor to recommend a dietitian. You also can contact the American Dietetic Association (see chapter 46 for their contact information.)

Excerpted and adapted from "Heart Healthy Eating," Office on Women's Health (www.womenshealth.gov), January 1, 2008, and "Sodium: The Facts," Centers for Disease Control and Prevention (CDC, www.cdc.gov), November 2009.

Chapter 31

Controlling High Blood Pressure

Blood pressure is the force your blood makes against the walls of your arteries. The pressure is highest when your heart pumps blood into your arteries—when it beats. It is lowest between heartbeats, when your heart relaxes. A doctor or nurse will write down your blood pressure as the higher number over the lower number. For instance, you could have a blood pressure of 110/70 (read as "110 over 70").

A blood pressure reading of 120/80 to 139/89 is considered prehypertension. This means you don't have high blood pressure now but are likely to develop it in the future. High blood pressure (the medical term is hypertension) is a blood pressure reading of 140/90 or higher. High blood pressure (HBP) is a serious condition that can lead to coronary heart disease, heart failure, stroke, kidney failure, and other health problems.

Years of high blood pressure can damage artery walls, causing them to become stiff and narrow. This includes the arteries carrying blood to the heart. As a result, your heart cannot get the blood it needs to work well. This can cause a heart attack. In addition, high blood pressure forces the heart to work harder to push blood through the blood vessels. Over time, this may lead the heart muscle to thicken and stiffen, which may interfere with its function.

Blood Pressure Numbers

Blood pressure numbers include systolic and diastolic pressures. Systolic blood pressure is the pressure when the heart beats while pumping blood. Diastolic blood pressure is the pressure when the heart is at rest between beats.

You will most often see blood pressure numbers written with the systolic number above or before the diastolic, such as 120/80 mmHg. (mmHg stands for millimeters of mercury—the units used to measure blood pressure.)

Table 31.1 shows normal numbers for adults. It also shows which numbers put you at greater risk for health problems. Blood pressure tends to go up and down, even in people who have normal blood pressure. If your numbers stay above normal most of the time, you're at risk. The ranges in the table apply to most adults (aged 18 and older) who don't have short-term serious illnesses.

Table 31.1. Categories for Blood Pressure Levels in Adults

Category	Systolic (top number)		Diastolic (bottom number)
Normal	Less than 120	*and*	Less than 80
Prehyper-tension	120–139	*or*	80–89
High blood pressure			
Stage 1	140–159	*or*	90–99
Stage 2	160 or higher	*or*	100 or higher

Note: All measurements are in mmHg, or millimeters of mercury.

All levels above 120/80 mmHg raise your risk, and the risk grows as blood pressure levels rise. Prehypertension means you're likely to end up with HBP unless you take steps to prevent it.

If you're being treated for HBP and have repeat readings in the normal range, your blood pressure is under control. However, you still have the condition. You should see your doctor and stay on treatment to keep your blood pressure under control.

Your systolic and diastolic numbers may not be in the same blood pressure category. In this case, the more severe category is the one you're in. For example, if your systolic number is 160 and your diastolic number is 80, you have stage 2 HBP. If your systolic number is 120 and your diastolic number is 95, you have stage 1 HBP.

Types of HBP

When HBP has no known cause, it may be called essential hypertension, primary hypertension, or idiopathic hypertension. When another condition causes HBP, it's sometimes called secondary high blood pressure or secondary hypertension.

In some cases of HBP, only the systolic blood pressure number is high. This condition is called isolated systolic hypertension (ISH). Many older adults have this condition. ISH can cause as much harm as HBP in which both numbers are too high.

Causes

Blood pressure tends to rise with age unless you take steps to prevent or control it.

Certain medical problems, such as chronic kidney disease, thyroid disease, and sleep apnea, may cause blood pressure to rise. Certain medicines, such as asthma medicines (for example, corticosteroids) and cold-relief products, also may raise blood pressure.

In some women, blood pressure can go up if they use birth control pills, become pregnant, or take hormone replacement therapy. Women taking birth control pills usually have a small rise in both systolic and diastolic blood pressures. If you already have high blood pressure and want to use birth control pills, make sure your doctor knows about your HBP. Talk to him or her about how often you should have your blood pressure checked and how to control it while taking the pill.

Taking hormones to reduce the symptoms of menopause can cause a small rise in systolic blood pressure. If you already have HBP and want to start using hormones, talk to your doctor about the risks and benefits. If you decide to take hormones, find out how to control your blood pressure and how often you should have it checked.

Risk Factors

Certain traits, conditions, or habits are known to raise the risk for HBP. These conditions are called risk factors.

Older Age

Blood pressure tends to rise with age. If you're a male older than 45 or a female older than 55, your risk for HBP is higher. Over half of all Americans aged 60 and older have HBP. Isolated systolic hypertension is the most common form of HBP in older adults. About two out of three people over age 60 who have HBP have ISH.

Race/Ethnicity

HBP can affect anyone. However, it occurs more often in African American adults than in Caucasian or Hispanic American adults. In relation to these groups, African Americans tend to get HBP earlier in life, often have more severe HBP, are more likely to be aware they have HBP and to get treatment, are less likely than Caucasians and about as likely as Hispanic Americans to achieve target control levels with HBP treatment, and have higher rates than Caucasians of premature death from HBP-related complications, such as coronary heart disease, stroke, and kidney failure.

HBP risks vary among different groups of Hispanic American adults. For instance, Puerto Rican American adults have higher rates of HBP-related death than all other Hispanic groups and Caucasians. But Cuban Americans have lower rates than Caucasians.

Overweight or Obesity

You're more likely to develop prehypertension or HBP if you're overweight or obese. Overweight is having extra body weight from muscle, bone, fat, and/or water. Obesity is having a high amount of extra body fat.

Gender

Fewer adult women than men have HBP. But younger women (aged 18–59) are more likely than men to be aware of and get treatment for HBP.

Women aged 60 and older are as likely as men to be aware of and treated for HBP. However, among treated women aged 60 and older, blood pressure control is lower than in men in the same age group.

Unhealthy Lifestyle Habits

A number of lifestyle habits can raise your risk for HBP, including eating too much sodium (salt), drinking too much alcohol, not getting enough potassium in your diet, not doing enough physical activity, and smoking,

Other Risk Factors

A family history of HBP raises your risk for the condition. Long-lasting stress also can put you at risk for HBP. You're also more likely to develop HBP if you have prehypertension.

Signs and Symptoms

High blood pressure itself usually has no symptoms. Rarely, headaches may occur. You can have HBP for years without knowing it. During this time, HBP can damage the heart, blood vessels, kidneys, and other parts of the body. Some people only learn they have HBP after the damage has caused problems, such as coronary heart disease, stroke, or kidney failure.

Complications

When blood pressure stays high over time, it can damage the body. HBP can cause the following problems:

- It can cause the heart to get larger or weaker, which may lead to heart failure. Heart failure is a condition in which the heart can't pump enough blood throughout the body.

- It can cause aneurysms to form in blood vessels. An aneurysm is an abnormal bulge or ballooning in the wall of an artery. Common spots for aneurysms are the main artery that carries blood from the heart to the body; the arteries in the brain, legs, and intestines; and the artery leading to the spleen.

- It can cause blood vessels in the kidney to narrow, which may cause kidney failure.

- It can cause arteries throughout the body to narrow in some places, which limits blood flow (especially to the heart, brain, kidneys, and legs). This can cause a heart attack, stroke, kidney failure, or amputation of part of the leg.

- It can cause blood vessels in the eyes to burst or bleed, which may lead to vision changes or blindness.

Treatment

High blood pressure is treated with lifestyle changes and medicine. Most people who have HBP will need lifelong treatment. Sticking to your treatment plan is important. It can prevent or delay the problems linked to HBP and help you live and stay active longer.

Goals of Treatment

The treatment goal for most adults is to get and keep blood pressure below 140/90 mmHg. For adults who have diabetes or chronic kidney disease, the goal is to get and keep blood pressure below 130/80 mmHg.

Healthy habits can help you control HBP. Healthy habits include following a healthy eating plan, doing enough physical activity, maintaining a healthy weight, quitting smoking, and managing and learning to cope with stress.

If you combine these measures, you can achieve even better results than taking single steps. Making lifestyle changes can be hard. Start by making one healthy lifestyle change and then adopt others.

Some people can control their blood pressure with lifestyle changes alone, but many people can't. Keep in mind that the main goal is blood pressure control. If your doctor prescribes medicine as part of your treatment plan, keep up your healthy habits. This will help you better control your blood pressure.

Ongoing Care

Go for medical checkups or tests as your doctor advises. Your doctor may need to change or add medicines to your treatment plan over time. Regular checkups allow your doctor to change your treatment right away if your blood pressure goes up again.

Keeping track of your blood pressure is vital. Have your blood pressure checked on the schedule your doctor advises. You may want to learn how to check your blood pressure at home. Your doctor can help you with this. Each time you check your own blood pressure, you should write down your numbers and the date.

During checkups, you can ask your doctor or health care team any questions you have about your lifestyle or medicine treatments.

Reviewed for currency and excerpted from "High Blood Pressure," National Heart, Lung, and Blood Institute (NHLBI, www.nhlbi.nih.gov), November 2008, with an excerpt from "Frequently Asked Questions about Heart Disease," Office on Women's Health (www.womenshealth.gov), February 2, 2009.

Chapter 32

Controlling High Cholesterol

Cholesterol, a waxy substance found in cells in all parts of the body, is a building block of our body's cells. It is made by the liver, and certain foods are an added source of cholesterol. We all need some cholesterol, but our bodies can make all the cholesterol we need. We also take in cholesterol from the food we eat. Many people have the right amount of cholesterol. Other people have too much. High cholesterol sometimes runs in families.

There are different types of cholesterol. The two main types are often called bad and good. Bad cholesterol can damage the heart and arteries, but good cholesterol does not cause damage.

Just having high cholesterol does not cause any symptoms. Most people do not know they have high cholesterol unless they get tested. Having a blood test to check your cholesterol will tell you if your levels are on target.

Bad Cholesterol (LDL Cholesterol)

Everyone should try to keep bad (low-density lipoprotein, or LDL) cholesterol as low as possible. If your doctor or nurse tells you you have high cholesterol, it means your bad cholesterol is too high.

When you have too much bad cholesterol in your blood, it can build up on the walls of your arteries. This buildup is called plaque. Plaque can narrow your arteries and make it harder for blood to flow. Plaque can lead to heart attacks and strokes. Keeping bad cholesterol at a low level can help avoid these problems.

Good Cholesterol (HDL Cholesterol)

Good (high-density lipoprotein, or HDL) cholesterol helps remove extra cholesterol from the body. When your good cholesterol is higher, your chance of heart disease is lower. A good cholesterol of 60 or higher helps protect against heart attacks and strokes.

Triglycerides

Triglycerides are a kind of fat found in your blood. The body makes triglycerides. They are also found in food. Your body needs this kind of fat, but it's best to keep your triglycerides low. Less than 150 is usually the goal.

Checking Cholesterol Levels

Cholesterol is measured by a blood test done at your doctor's office or a lab. A cholesterol test will tell you your total cholesterol level. It will also tell you the levels of your good and bad cholesterol and your triglycerides.

How often you have this blood test may depend on your personal risk for heart attack or stroke. Talk to your doctor or nurse about how often your cholesterol should be checked.

Your health care provider can help you set a goal for your cholesterol. The target for your bad cholesterol depends on your risk factors for heart disease. Risk factors are things that increase your chance of having a heart attack or stroke. If you have more risk factors, your doctor or nurse will recommend a lower target for your bad cholesterol. Talk with your doctor or nurse about setting your cholesterol goal.

Treatment

The first step in controlling your cholesterol is to eat a balanced diet and be more active. Even small changes can make a big difference. Your doctor or nurse may recommend a special cholesterol-lowering diet.

Some people can reach their cholesterol goals by eating a balanced diet and exercising. But many people will also need medicine to lower their cholesterol.

Talking with Your Doctor

Everyone with high cholesterol should be on a cholesterol-lowering diet. Exercising can help, too. If you can't get to your cholesterol goal with diet and exercise alone, you may need to start a cholesterol medicine. Chapter 19 details the medicines most frequently used to manage blood cholesterol. Work with your doctor or nurse to set up a plan that works for you.

Excerpted and adapted from "Treating High Cholesterol: A Guide for Adults," Agency for Healthcare Research and Quality (AHRQ, www.ahrq.gov), November 18, 2009, with an excerpt from "Frequently Asked Questions about Heart Disease," Office on Women's Health (www.womenshealth.gov), February 2, 2009.

Chapter 33

Controlling Diabetes

Heart disease is a major complication of diabetes and the leading cause of early death among people with diabetes—about 65% of people with diabetes die from heart disease and stroke. Here are some facts about heart disease and diabetes:

- Adults with diabetes are two to four times more likely to have heart disease or suffer a stroke than people without diabetes.

- High blood glucose in adults with diabetes increases the risk for heart attack, stroke, angina, and coronary artery disease.

- People with type 2 diabetes also have high rates of high blood pressure, lipid problems, and obesity that contribute to their high rates of heart disease.

- Smoking doubles the risk of heart disease in people with diabetes.

Controlling the multiple risk factors associated with heart disease can reduce illness and death in people with diabetes.

Comprehensive control of diabetes involves optimal management of A1C (a measure of average blood glucose), blood pressure, and cholesterol. The ABC treatment goals for most people with diabetes are the following:

- **A:** A1C (blood glucose) less than 7%

- **B:** Blood pressure less than 130/80 millimeters of mercury (mmHg)

- **C:** Cholesterol—low-density lipoprotein (LDL)—less than 100 milligrams per deciliter (mg/dL)

The A1C Test

The A1C test (pronounced A-one-C) is a simple lab test that reflects your average blood glucose level over the previous three months. It is the best way to know your overall blood glucose control during this period of time. This test used to be called hemoglobin A1c or HbA1c. A small blood sample to check your A1C can be taken at any time of day.

You and your health care team should discuss the A1C goal that is right for you. Most people with diabetes have an A1C goal of less than 7. An A1C higher than 7 means you have a greater chance of eye disease, kidney disease, or nerve damage. Lowering your A1C—by any amount—can improve your chances of staying healthy.

Benefits

Research studies and clinical trials have demonstrated the following benefits of optimal control of the ABCs of diabetes:

- Intensive glucose control reduces the risk of any heart disease event by 42% and the risk of heart attack, stroke, or death from heart disease by 57%.

- In general, every percentage point drop in A1C blood test results (e.g., from 8% to 7%) reduces the risk of diabetes and kidney, eye, and nerve disease by 40%.

- Blood pressure control reduces the risk of heart disease among persons with diabetes by 33% to 50% and the risk of diabetic kidney, eye, and nerve disease by approximately 33%. In general, for every 10-mmHg reduction in systolic blood pressure, the risk for any complication related to diabetes is reduced by 12%.

- Improved control of cholesterol or blood lipids (for example, high-density lipoprotein [HDL], LDL, and triglycerides) can reduce heart disease complications by 20% to 50%.

National surveys of people with diabetes show there still is a wide gap between current and desired diabetes care as evidenced by the following facts:

- Only 7.3% of people surveyed were at goal for all three ABCs of diabetes.

- Two in five have poorly controlled LDL cholesterol.

- One in three has poorly controlled blood pressure.

- One in five has poorly controlled blood glucose.

Take Action

People with diabetes can work with their health care team to develop and use an action plan to reach their ABC goals. An action plan can help people do the following:

- Reach and stay at a healthy weight. Being overweight or obese is a risk factor for heart attack and stroke.

- Get at least 30 to 60 minutes of physical activity. Brisk walking or a similar activity most days of the week can help with weight loss and lower blood pressure.

- Eat foods that are low in saturated fats, trans fats, cholesterol, salt (sodium), and added sugars—choose lean meats, poultry, fish, nuts (in small amounts), and fat-free or low-fat milk products.

- Eat more fiber—whole grains, fruits, vegetables, and dry peas and beans.

- Stop smoking—or ask a health care team member for help quitting. Smoking is one of the major risk factors associated with heart attack and stroke.

- Take medications as directed—and ask a doctor about taking daily aspirin.

- Ask family and friends for help managing diabetes. This support can help people reach their goals.

Reviewed for currency and excerpted from "The Link between Diabetes and Cardiovascular Disease," National Diabetes Education Program (NDEP, www .ndep.nih.gov), February 2007. Supplemental information about the A1C test is adapted from "If You Have Diabetes, Know Your Blood Sugar Numbers," NDEP, July 2005.

Chapter 34

Managing Your Weight

If you have heart disease and are overweight or obese (extremely overweight), your risks of heart attack and other heart complications rise sharply. This is true even if you have no other risk factors.

Being overweight or obese also increases your chances of developing other major risk factors for heart disease and heart attack, such as diabetes, high blood pressure, and high blood cholesterol. Overall, obese people are more likely to die of heart disease than normal-weight individuals. The bottom line: maintaining a healthy weight is a necessary part of controlling heart disease.

Energy Balance

If you need to lose weight, here's some good news: a small weight loss—just 5% to 10% of your current weight—can help lower the risks of heart attack and other serious medical disorders. The best way to take off pounds is to do so gradually by getting more physical activity and eating a balanced diet lower in calories and fat. For some people at very high risk, medication also may be necessary.

To develop a weight-loss or weight-maintenance program that works well for you, consult your doctor, registered dietitian, or qualified nutritionist.

A person's weight is the result of many things—height, genes, metabolism, behavior, and environment. Maintaining a healthy weight requires keeping a balance of energy. You must balance the calories you get from food and beverages with the calories you use keeping your body going and being physically active. If the same amount of energy comes in and goes out over time, then weight stays the same. If more energy comes in than goes out over time, the result is weight gain. If more energy goes out than in over time, the result is weight loss.

Your energy in and out don't have to balance exactly every day. It's the balance over time that will help you maintain a healthy weight in the long run. For many people, this balance means eating fewer calories and increasing physical activity.

Facts about Weight Loss

We have all heard the facts: to lose weight, you have to eat less and move more. But this is often easier said than done. Many people make repeated attempts—often using different fad diets and weight loss gimmicks—and are unsuccessful.

Did you know that a reasonable and safe weight loss is one to two pounds per week? While it may take as long as six months to lose weight in this manner, it will make it easier to keep the weight off. And it will give you the time to make new healthy lifestyle changes such as eating a healthy diet and increasing your physical activity level.

Did you know it is better to maintain a moderate weight loss over a longer period of time than it is to lose lots of weight and regain it? You can consider additional weight loss after you have lost 10% of your current body weight and have maintained it for six months.

To be successful at losing weight, you need to adopt a new life-style. This means making changes such as eating healthy foods, be-ing more physically active, and learning how to change behaviors. Over time, these changes will become routine. But there are some people for whom lifestyle changes don't work no matter how hard they try. Weight-loss medications and weight-loss surgery can be options for these people if they are at increased risk from over-weight or obesity.

Daily Calorie Intake

To lose weight, most people need to cut down on the number of calories (units of energy) they get from food and beverages and increase their physical activity. For a weight loss of one to two pounds per week, daily intake should be reduced by 500 to 1,000 calories. In general, the following guidelines apply:

- Eating plans containing 1,000–1,200 calories will help most women lose weight safely.

- Eating plans between 1,200 calories and 1,600 calories each day are suitable for men and may also be appropri-ate for women who weigh 165 pounds or more or who exercise regularly.

- If you are on a 1,600-calorie diet but do not lose weight, you may want to try a 1,200-calorie diet.

If you are hungry on either diet, you may want to boost your calo-ries by 100 to 200 per day. Very low calorie diets of less than 800 calories each day should not be used routinely because they re-quire special monitoring by a doctor.

Portion and Serving Sizes

A portion is the amount of a food you choose to eat for a meal or snack. It can be big or small—you decide. A serving is a measured amount of food or drink, such as one slice of bread or one cup of milk. Some foods most people consume as a single serving actually contain multiple servings (for example, a 20-ounce soda or a 3-ounce bag of chips).

Nutrition recommendations use serving sizes to help people know how much of different types of foods they should eat to get the nutrients they need. The Nutrition Facts label on packaged foods also lists a serving size. The serving sizes on packaged foods are not always the same as those included in nutrition recommendations. However, serving sizes are standardized to make it easier to compare similar foods.

Read labels as you shop. Pay attention to the serving size and the servings per container. All labels list total calories and fat in a serving size of the product. Compare the total calories in the product you choose with others like it; choose the one lowest in calories and fat.

Food Preparation

One way to control calories is to prepare low-calorie, low-fat foods. It is important to learn how certain ingredients can add unwanted calories and fat to low-fat dishes—making them no longer lower in calories or fat. The following list provides examples of lower-fat cooking methods and tips on how to serve your low-fat dishes.

Low-Fat Cooking Methods

These cooking methods tend to be lower in fat:

- Baking
- Broiling
- Microwaving
- Roasting—vegetables and/or chicken without skin
- Steaming
- Lightly stir-frying or sautéing in cooking spray, small amounts of vegetable oil, or reduced sodium broth
- Grilling seafood, chicken, or vegetables

Low-Fat Flavorings

Here is a list of low-fat flavorings you can add during preparation or at the table:

- Herbs—including oregano, basil, cilantro, thyme, parsley, sage, or rosemary
- Spices—including cinnamon, nutmeg, pepper, or paprika
- Reduced fat or fat-free salad dressing
- Mustard
- Ketchup
- Fat-free mayonnaise
- Fat-free or reduced fat sour cream
- Fat-free or reduced fat yogurt
- Reduced sodium soy sauce
- Salsa
- Lemon or lime juice
- Vinegar
- Horseradish
- Fresh ginger
- Sprinkled buttered flavor (not made with real butter)
- Red pepper flakes
- Sprinkle of parmesan cheese (stronger flavor than most cheese)
- Sodium-free salt substitute
- Jelly or fruit preserves on toast or bagels

Dining Out

You can eat healthy food when dining out or bringing food home if you know how.

You are the customer. Ask for what you want. Most restaurants will honor your requests. Ask questions. Don't be intimidated by the menu—your server will be able to tell you how foods are prepared or suggest substitutions on the menu.

To reduce portion sizes, try ordering appetizers as your main meal or share an entrée with a friend or family member.

Limiting your calories and fat can be easy as long as you know what to order. Try asking these questions when you call ahead or before you order. Ask the restaurant whether they would, on request, serve fat-free (skim) milk rather than whole milk or cream; reveal the type of cooking oil used; trim visible fat off poultry or meat; leave all butter, gravy, or sauces off a side dish or entrée; serve salad dressing on the side; or accommodate special requests if made in advance by telephone or in person.

Look for terms such as "steamed in its own juice" (au jus), "garden fresh," "broiled," "baked," "roasted," "poached," "tomato juice," "dry boiled" (in wine or lemon juice), or "lightly sautéed."

Be aware of foods high in calories, fat, and saturated fat. Watch out for terms such as "butter sauce," "fried," "crispy," "creamed," "in cream or cheese sauce," "au gratin," "au fromage," "escalloped," "parmesan," "hollandaise," "béarnaise," "marinated (in oil)," "stewed," "basted," "sautéed," "stir-fried," "casserole," "hash," "prime," "pot pie," and "pastry crust."

Fast Food

When you eat in a heart-healthy way, you don't have to give up eating fast food completely. You can eat right and still eat fast food if you select carefully. Here are some tips on fast foods to choose:

- Order a small hamburger instead of a larger one. Try the lower fat hamburger. Hold the extra sauce.

- Order roast beef for a leaner choice than most burgers.

- Order a baked potato instead of french fries. Be careful of high-fat toppings like sour cream, butter, or cheese.

- Order grilled, broiled, or baked fish or chicken.

- Order skim or 1% milk instead of a milkshake. Try the low-fat frozen yogurt or low-fat milkshake.

- Order a salad. Use vinegar and oil or low-calorie dressing.

- Create a salad at the salad bar. Choose any raw vegetables, fruits, or beans. Limit toppings high in saturated fat such as cheese, fried noodles, and bacon bits as well as some salads made with mayonnaise. Also limit salad dressings high in saturated fat and cholesterol.

- For sandwich toppings try lettuce, tomato, onion, mustard, and ketchup instead of toppings high in saturated fat, such as cheese, bacon, special sauces, or butter.

- Order pizza with vegetable toppings such as peppers, mushrooms, or onions instead of extra cheese, pepperoni, or sausage.

Weight-Loss Programs

The best way to reach a healthy weight is to follow a sensible eating plan and engage in regular physical activity. Weight-loss programs should encourage healthy behaviors that help you lose weight and that you can maintain over time.

Safe and effective weight-loss programs should include the following:

- Healthy eating plans that reduce calories but do not rule out specific foods or food groups

- Regular physical activity and/or exercise instruction

- Tips on healthy behavior changes that also consider your cultural needs

- Slow and steady weight loss of about one to two pounds per week and not more than three pounds per week (weight loss may be faster at the start of a program)

- Medical care if you are planning to lose weight by following a special formula diet, such as a very low-calorie diet

- A plan to keep the weight off after you have lost it

If you decide to join any kind of weight-loss program, here are some questions to ask in advance:

- Is the diet safe? The eating plan should be low in calories but still provide all the nutrients needed to stay healthy, including vitamins and minerals.

- Does the program provide counseling to help you change your eating, activity, and personal habits? The program should teach you how to change permanently those eating habits and lifestyle factors, such as lack of physical activity, that have contributed to weight gain.

- Is the staff made up of a variety of qualified counselors and health professionals such as nutritionists, registered dietitians, doctors, nurses, psychologists, and exercise physiologists? You need to be evaluated by a physician if you have any health problems, are currently taking any medicine, or plan to lose more than 15–20 pounds. If your weight control plan uses a very low-calorie diet (a special liquid formula that replaces all food for one to four months), an exam and follow-up visits by a doctor are also needed.

- Is training available on how to deal with times when you may feel stressed and slip back to old habits? The program should provide long-term strategies to deal with weight problems you may have in the future. These strategies might include setting up a support system and establishing a physical activity routine.

- Is attention paid to keeping the weight off? How long is this phase? Choose a program that teaches skills and techniques to make permanent changes in eating habits and levels of physical activity to prevent weight gain.

- Are food choices flexible and suitable?

- Are weight goals set by the client and the health professional? The program should consider your food likes and dislikes and your lifestyle when your weight-loss goals are planned.

There are other questions you can ask about how well a program works. Because many programs don't gather this information, you may not get answers. But it's still important to ask the following:

- What percentage of people completes the program?

- What is the average weight loss among people who finish the program?

- What percentage of people maintains their weight loss after one, two, and even five years?

- What percentage of people has problems or side effects? What are they?

- Are there fees or costs for additional items such as dietary supplements?

Remember, quick weight-loss methods don't provide lasting results. Weight-loss methods that rely on diet aids like drinks, prepackaged foods, or diet pills don't work in the long run.

Calculating Your Body Mass Index

Body mass index (BMI) is a measure of body fat based on height and weight that applies to adult men and women. You can compute your BMI using the National Heart, Lung, and Blood Institute's online calculator at www.nhlbisupport.com/bmi.

Weight-Loss Medications

Weight-loss drugs approved by the Food and Drug Administration (FDA) may be an option for some patients and should be used only as part of a program that includes diet, physical activity, and behavioral changes.

Weight-loss drugs may be considered in the following instances:

- For people with a body mass index greater than or equal to 27 who also have obesity-related risk factors or diseases

- For people with a BMI greater than or equal to 30 without other obesity-related risk factors or diseases

- If weight loss of one pound per week has not occurred after six months of a calorie-controlled diet and physical activity

Two weight-loss drugs have been approved by the FDA. They are sibutramine (Meridia®) and orlistat (Xenical®). These drugs have been shown to produce a modest weight loss (between 4.4 and 22 pounds), although some people lose more weight. It is not possible to predict exactly how much weight an individual may lose. Most of the weight loss occurs within the first six months of therapy.

People with high blood pressure, congestive heart failure, arrhythmias, or a history of stroke should not take sibutramine because it causes an increase in heart rate and blood pressure.

If you think you're a candidate for weight-loss drugs, you should discuss this option with your doctor.

Patients on weight-loss drugs need to be monitored for side effects by their doctors. Follow-up visits are generally recommended within two to four weeks after starting the medication, then monthly for three months, then every three months for the first year after starting the medication. After the first year, your doctor will advise you on appropriate return visits. The purpose of these visits is to monitor weight, blood pressure, and pulse; discuss side effects; conduct laboratory tests; and answer your questions.

Weight-Loss Surgery

Weight-loss surgery may be an option for patients with severe obesity (BMI greater than or equal to 40 or BMI greater than or equal to 35 with high-risk, comorbid conditions such as life-threatening severe sleep apnea, obesity-related cardiomyopathy, or severe diabetes). Weight-loss surgery may also be considered for people with severe obesity when other methods of treatment have failed.

Two types of operations have proven effective. One is a banded gastroplasty that limits the amount of food and liquid the stomach can hold. The other is a Roux-en-Y gastric bypass that, in addition to limiting food intake, also alters digestion.

Both these procedures carry a risk of complications depending on the individual's weight and overall health. Lifelong medical monitoring is necessary as well as a comprehensive program before and after surgery to provide guidance on diet, physical activity, and psychosocial concerns.

If you feel you are a candidate for weight-loss surgery, talk to your doctor. Ask him or her to assess whether you are a candidate for the surgery and discuss the risks, benefits, and what to expect.

Meeting Long-Term Challenges

Weight management is a long-term challenge influenced by behavioral, emotional, and physical factors. Changing the way you approach weight loss can help you be more successful. Most people who try to lose weight focus on one thing: weight loss. However, setting goals and focusing on physical activity changes is much more productive.

Set the Right Goals

Setting the right goals is an important first step. Did you know that the amount of weight loss needed to improve health might be much less than you want to lose to look thinner? If your provider

327

suggests an initial weight-loss goal that still seems too heavy, please understand that your health can be greatly improved by a loss of 5% to 10% of your starting weight. This doesn't mean you have to stop there, but it does mean that an initial goal of 5% to 10% of your starting weight is both realistic and valuable.

It's important to set diet and/or physical activity goals. People who are successful at managing their weight set only two to three goals at a time.

Effective goals are specific, realistic, and forgiving (less than perfect). For example: "Exercise more" is a fine goal, but it's not specific enough. "Walk five miles every day" is specific and measurable, but is it achievable if you're just starting out? "Walk 30 minutes every day" is more attainable, but what happens if you're held up at work one day and there's a thunderstorm during your walking time on another day? "Walk 30 minutes, five days each week" is specific, achievable, and forgiving. It's a great goal.

Shaping

Shaping is a technique where you set some short-term goals that get you closer and closer to the ultimate goal (for example, reduce your fat intake from 40% of your total calories to 35% of your calories, and ultimately to 30%). It is based on the concept that nothing succeeds like success.

Shaping uses two important behavioral principles: continuous goals that move you ahead in small steps to reach a distant point and continuous rewards to keep you motivated to make changes.

Reward Success

Rewards you control can encourage achievement of your goals, especially ones that have been hard to reach. An effective reward is something desirable, timely, and dependent upon meeting your goal. The rewards you choose may be material (for example, a movie, music CD, or a payment toward buying a larger item) or acts of self-kindness (for example, an afternoon off from work, a massage, or personal time). Frequent small rewards earned for meeting smaller goals are more effective than bigger rewards requiring a long, difficult effort.

Self-Monitoring

Self-monitoring refers to observing and recording some aspect of your behavior—such as calorie intake, servings of fruits and vegetables eaten, or amount of physical activity—or an outcome of these behaviors, such as weight. Self-monitoring of a behavior can be used at times when you're not sure how you are doing and times when you want the behavior to improve. Self-monitoring of a behavior usually moves you closer to the desired behavior. When you record your behavior, you produce real-time records for you and your health care provider to discuss. For example, keeping a record of your activity can let you and your provider quickly know how you are doing. When your record shows your activity is increasing, you'll be encouraged to keep it up.

Regular monitoring of your weight is key to keeping it off. Remember these four points if you are keeping a weight chart or graph:

- One day's diet and activity routine won't necessarily affect your weight the next day. Your weight will change quite a bit over the course of a few days because of fluctuations in water and body fat.

- Try to weigh yourself at a set time once or twice per week. It can be when you first wake up and before eating and drinking, after exercise, or right before dinner.

- Whatever time you choose, just make sure it is always the same time and use the same scale to help you keep the most accurate records.

- It may also be helpful to create a graph of your weight as a visual reminder of how you're doing, rather than just listing numbers.

Control Cues

Stimulus (cue) control involves learning what social or environmental cues encourage undesired eating and then changing those cues. For example, you may learn from your self-monitoring techniques or from sessions with your health care provider that you're more likely to overeat when watching TV, when treats are on display by the office coffee pot, or when around a certain friend.

Ways to change the situation include the following:

- Separating the association of eating from the cue (don't eat while watching television)

- Avoiding or eliminating the cue (leave the coffee room immediately after pouring coffee)

- Changing the environment (plan to meet this friend in a nonfood setting)

In general, visible and reachable food items often lead to unplanned eating.

Change Habits

Changing the way you eat can help you eat less and not feel deprived.

- Eating slowly will help you feel satisfied when you've eaten the right amount of food for you. It takes 15 or more minutes for your brain to get the message you've been fed. Slowing your rate of eating can allow you to feel full sooner and, therefore, help you eat less.

- Eating lots of vegetables and fruits and also starting a meal with a broth-based soup can help you feel fuller.

- Using smaller plates helps moderate portions so they don't appear too small.

- Drinking at least eight glasses of noncaloric beverages each day will help you feel full, will help you possibly eat less, and may benefit you in other ways.

- Serving food from the kitchen instead of at the table can help you be less tempted to eat more.

- Pouring food or snacks from large packages into smaller ones and keeping them in your cupboard can prevent overeating.

Weight Maintenance

Once you've reached your weight-loss goal, maintaining your lower body weight can be a challenge.

Successful weight maintenance is defined as a weight regain of less than six to seven pounds in two years and a sustained lowered waist circumference reduction of least two inches. The key to weight maintenance is to continue the healthy lifestyle changes you have adopted. Staying on a healthy diet and aiming for 60–90 minutes of physical activity most days of the week will help you maintain your lower weight. For long-term motivation, ask for encouragement from your health care provider and friends or family via telephone or e-mail or join a support group. The longer you can maintain your weight, the better your chances for overall long-term success in weight reduction.

Reviewed for currency and excerpted from "Your Guide to Living Well with Heart Disease," November 2005, "Aim for a Healthy Weight," August 2005, and "Calculate Your Body Mass Index," 2010, all three produced by the National Heart, Lung, and Blood Institute (NHLBI, www.nhlbi.nih.gov).

Chapter 35

Quitting Smoking

Smoking is the leading cause of preventable death and disease in the United States, according to the Centers for Disease Control and Prevention. If you have heart disease and continue to smoke, your risk of having a heart attack is very high. If you live or work with others, your second-hand smoke can cause them numerous health problems—including a higher risk of heart attack—even if they don't smoke themselves. By the same token, if you have heart disease and live or work with someone who smokes, your own risk of heart attack goes up considerably.

Smoking puts stress on the heart in many ways. The nicotine in cigarettes constricts the coronary arteries, which raises blood pressure and forces the heart to work harder. Smoking also raises carbon monoxide levels and reduces oxygen levels in the blood. It's a double whammy: smoking both increases the heart's need for oxygen and restricts the amount of oxygen it receives.

There is simply no safe way to smoke. Low-tar and low-nicotine cigarettes do not lessen the risks of a heart attack. The only safe and healthful course is not to smoke at all.

Reasons to Quit

There are numerous reasons to quit smoking. Quitting smoking will immediately and significantly reduce your risk of further heart disease complications. After a few days—once nicotine and carbon monoxide are cleared from your body—your blood pressure will go down, and the levels of oxygen and carbon monoxide in your blood can return to normal. Within one year after quitting, your blood flow and breathing will be improved and your coughing and shortness of breath will be reduced.

Here are some other reasons:

- You will feel better.

- You will have more energy and breathe easier.

- Your chances of getting sick will go down.

- Smoking is dangerous. More than 435,000 Americans die each year from smoking.

- If you are pregnant, your baby will be healthier. Your baby will get more oxygen.

- The people around you, especially children, will be healthier. Breathing in other people's smoke can cause asthma and other health problems.

- You will have more money. If you smoke one pack per day, quitting smoking could save you up to $150 a month. If you smoke two packs, you'll save $300 per month. If you smoke three packs daily, quitting could save you $450 per month.

How to Quit

Some people prefer to quit on their own, while others find group support helpful. When it comes to quitting smoking, a combination of strategies usually works best.

Set a Quit Date

Set a quit date, and don't smoke after the date you pick. Change the things around you—for example, get rid of all cigarettes and ash-trays in your home, car, and place of work, and do not let people smoke in your home. After you quit, don't smoke—not even a puff. Don't use any tobacco.

Take Medicine

Also consider using a medicine to help you stay off cigarettes. Some medications contain very small amounts of nicotine, which can help lessen the urge to smoke. They include nicotine gum (available over the counter), a nicotine patch (available over the counter and by prescription), a nicotine inhaler (by prescription only), and a nicotine nasal spray (by prescription only). Another quitting aid is bupropion SR, a medicine that contains no nicotine but reduces the craving for cigarettes. It is available only by prescription. Varenicline (Chantix®) is another prescription medication that can help with quitting smoking. While all these medications can help people quit smoking, they are not safe for everyone. Talk with your doctor about whether you should try any of these medicines.

You can buy nicotine gum, the nicotine patch, or the nicotine lozenge at a drugstore. You can ask your pharmacist for more information. Most health insurance will pay for these medicines.

Get Support

Tell your family, friends, and the people you work with that you are going to quit. Ask for their support. Talk to your doctor, nurse, or other health care worker. They can help you quit.

Call 800-QUIT-NOW (800-784-8669) to be connected to the quitline in your state. It's free. They will set up a quit plan with you.

A number of free or low-cost programs are available to help people stop smoking. They include classes offered by local chapters of the

American Lung Association and the American Cancer Society. Other low-cost programs can be found through hospitals, health maintenance organizations (HMOs), workplaces, and community groups.

Stay Quit

If you slip and smoke or chew tobacco, don't give up. Try again soon. Set a new quit date to get back on track. Avoid alcohol. Avoid being around smoking. Eat healthy food and get exercise. Keep a positive attitude. You can do it.

Most people try several times before they quit for good. Quitting is hard, but you can quit.

Excerpted and adapted from "Your Guide to Living Well with Heart Disease," National Heart, Lung, and Blood Institute (NHLBI, www.nhlbi.nih.gov), November 2005, and "Help for Smokers and Other Tobacco Users," Agency for Healthcare Research and Quality (AHRQ, www.ahrq.gov), May 2008.

Chapter 36

Managing Stress

Stress is a feeling you get when faced with a challenge. In small doses, stress can be good for you because it makes you more alert and gives you a burst of energy. For instance, if you start to cross the street and see a car about to run you over, the jolt you feel helps you jump out of the way before you get hit. But feeling stressed for a long time can take a toll on your mental and physical health, and long-term stress can worsen heart disease. Even though it may seem hard to find ways to de-stress with all the other things you have to do to manage your heart disease, it's important to find those ways. Your health depends on it.

Causes

Stress happens when people feel they don't have the tools to manage all the demands in their lives. Stress can be short-term or long-term. Missing the bus or arguing with your spouse or partner can cause short-term stress. Money problems or trouble at work can cause long-term stress. Even happy events, like having a baby or getting married, can cause stress. Some of the most common stressful life events include the death of a spouse, the death of a close family member, divorce, losing your job, a major personal illness or injury, marital separation, marriage, pregnancy, retirement, and spending time in jail.

Signs and Symptoms

Everyone responds to stress a little differently. Your symptoms may be different from someone else's. Here are some of the signs to look for:

- Not eating or eating too much
- Feeling you have no control
- Needing to have too much control
- Forgetfulness
- Headaches
- Lack of energy
- Lack of focus
- Trouble getting things done
- Poor self-esteem
- Short temper
- Trouble sleeping
- Upset stomach
- Back pain
- General aches and pains

These symptoms may also be signs of depression or anxiety, which can be caused by long-term stress.

Impact on Health

The body responds to stress by releasing stress hormones. These hormones make blood pressure, heart rate, and blood sugar levels go up. Long-term stress can contribute to a variety of health problems, including mental health disorders like depression and anxiety, obesity, heart disease, high blood pressure, abnormal heart beats, menstrual problems, and acne and other skin problems.

Handling Stress

Everyone has to deal with stress. There are steps you can take to help you handle stress in a positive way and keep it from making you sick. Try these tips to keep stress in check.

Develop a New Attitude

- Become a problem solver. Make a list of the things that cause you stress. From your list, figure out which problems you can solve now and which are beyond your control for the moment. From your list of problems that you can solve now, start with the little ones. Learn how to calmly look at a problem, think of possible solutions, and take action to solve the problem. Being able to solve small problems will give you confidence to tackle the big ones. And feeling confident that you can solve problems will go a long way to helping you feel less stressed.

- Be flexible. Sometimes it's not worth the stress to argue. Give in once in awhile or meet people halfway.

- Get organized. Think ahead about how you're going to spend your time. Write a to-do list. Figure out what's most important and do those things first.

- Set limits. When it comes to things like work and family, figure out what you can really do. There are only so many hours in the day. Set limits for yourself and others. Don't be afraid to say no to requests for your time and energy.

Relax

- Take deep breaths. If you're feeling stressed, taking a few deep breaths makes you breathe slower and helps your muscles relax.

- Stretch. Stretching can also help relax your muscles and make you feel less tense.

- Massage tense muscles. Having someone massage the muscles in the back of your neck and upper back can help you feel less tense.

- Take time to do something you want to do. We all have lots of things we have to do. But often we don't take the time to do the things we really want to do. It could be listening to music, reading a good book, or going to a movie. Think of this as an order from your doctor so you won't feel guilty.

Take Care of Your Body

- Get enough sleep. Getting enough sleep helps you recover from the stresses of the day. Also, being well rested helps you think better so you are prepared to handle problems as they come up. Most adults need seven to nine hours of sleep a night to feel rested.

- Eat right. Try to fuel up with fruits, vegetables, beans, and whole grains. Don't be fooled by the jolt you get from caffeine or high-sugar snack foods. Your energy will wear off, and you could wind up feeling more tired than you did before.

- Get moving. Getting physical activity can not only help relax your tense muscles but can also improve your mood. Research shows that physical activity can help relieve symptoms of depression and anxiety.

- Don't deal with stress in unhealthy ways, including drinking too much alcohol, using drugs, smoking, or overeating.

Connect with Others

- Share your stress. Talking about your problems with friends or family members can sometimes help you feel better. They might also help you see your problems in a new way and suggest novel solutions.

- Get help from a professional if you need it. If you feel you can no longer cope, talk to your doctor. She or he may suggest counseling to help you learn better ways to deal with stress. Your doctor may also prescribe medicine, such as antidepressants or sleep aids.

- Help others. Volunteering in your community can help you make new friends and feel better about yourself.

Excerpted and adapted from "Stress and Your Health," Office on Women's Health (www.womenshealth.gov), March 17, 2010.

Chapter 37

Your Ongoing Health Care Needs

Heart Disease

Heart disease can cause serious complications. However, if you follow your doctor's advice and change your habits, you can prevent or reduce your chances of dying suddenly from heart problems, having a heart attack and permanently damaging your heart muscle, damaging your heart because of reduced oxygen supply, and having arrhythmias (irregular heartbeats).

Ongoing Care

Doing physical activity regularly, taking prescribed medicine, following a heart-healthy eating plan, and watching your weight can help control heart disease.

See your doctor regularly to keep track of your blood pressure and blood cholesterol and blood sugar levels. A cholesterol blood test will show your levels of LDL cholesterol, HDL cholesterol, and triglycerides. A fasting blood glucose test will check your blood sugar level and show if you're at risk for or have diabetes. These tests will show whether you need more treatments for your heart disease.

Talk to your doctor about how often you should schedule office visits or blood tests. Between those visits, call your doctor if you develop any new symptoms or if your symptoms worsen.

Anxiety or Depression

You may feel depressed or anxious if you've been diagnosed with heart disease and/or had a heart attack. You may worry about heart problems or making lifestyle changes that are necessary for your health. Your doctor may recommend medicine, professional counseling, or relaxation therapy if you have depression or anxiety.

Physical activity can improve mental well-being, but you should talk to your doctor before starting any fitness activities. It's important to treat any anxiety or depression that develops because it raises your risk of having a heart attack.

Heart Attack

Many people survive heart attacks and live active and full lives. If you get help quickly, treatment can limit the damage to your heart muscle. Less heart damage improves your chances for a better quality of life after a heart attack.

Ongoing Care

After a heart attack, you will need treatment for heart disease to prevent another heart attack. Your doctor may recommend lifestyle changes, such as quitting smoking, following a healthy diet, increasing your physical activity, and losing weight, if needed. Your doctor may also prescribe medicine to control chest pain or discomfort, blood pressure, blood cholesterol, and your heart's workload. Participation in a cardiac rehabilitation program may help you improve your quality of life.

Returning to Normal Activities

After a heart attack, most people without chest pain or discomfort or other complications can safely return to most of their normal activities within a few weeks. Most can begin walking immediately. Sexual activity also can begin within a few weeks for most patients. Discuss with your doctor a safe schedule for returning to your normal activities, such as driving.

Anxiety and Depression

After a heart attack, many people worry about having another heart attack. Sometimes they feel depressed and have trouble adjusting to the new lifestyle required to limit further heart trouble. Your doctor may recommend medicine or professional counseling if you have depression or anxiety. Physical activity can improve mental well-being, but you should consult with your doctor before starting any fitness activities.

Arrhythmia

It's common to have an occasional extra heartbeat and not even be aware of it or to only have mild palpitations. People who have harmless arrhythmias can live healthy lives and usually don't need treatment for their arrhythmias. Even people who have serious arrhythmias often are treated successfully and lead normal lives.

Ongoing Care

If you have an arrhythmia that requires treatment, you should do the following:

- Keep all of your medical appointments. Always bring all medicines you're taking to all of your doctor visits. This helps ensure all your doctors know exactly what medicines you're taking, which can help prevent medication errors.

- Follow your doctor's instructions for taking medicines. Check with your doctor before taking over-the-counter medicines, nutritional supplements, or cold and allergy medicines.

- Tell your doctor if you're having side effects from your medicines. Side effects could include depression and palpitations. These side effects often can be treated.

- Tell your doctor if arrhythmia symptoms are getting worse or if you have new symptoms.

- Allow your doctor to check you regularly if you're taking blood-thinning medicines.

If you have an arrhythmia, taking care of yourself is important. If you feel dizzy or faint, you should lie down. Don't try to walk or drive. Let your doctor know about these symptoms.

Ask your doctor whether vagal maneuvers are an option for you. These exercises, which people who have certain arrhythmias can do, may help stop a rapid heartbeat.

Learn how to take your pulse. Discuss with your doctor what pulse rate is normal for you. Keep a record of changes in your pulse rate and share this information with your doctor.

Lifestyle Changes

Many arrhythmias are caused by underlying heart disease. Keep your heart healthy by following a healthy diet.

A healthy lifestyle also includes doing physical activity regularly, quitting smoking, maintaining a healthy weight, and keeping your blood cholesterol and blood pressure at healthy levels.

Strong emotional stress or anger can lead to arrhythmias. Try to manage stress and anger through activities such as yoga, quiet time, meditation, and relaxation techniques. Getting support from friends and family also can help you manage stress.

Your doctor may want you to avoid certain substances if they make your heart beat too fast. These substances may include alcohol and cold and cough medicines.

Excerpted and adapted from "Coronary Artery Disease," February 2009, "Heart Attack," March 2008, and "Arrhythmia," July 2009, all three produced by the National Heart, Lung, and Blood Institute (NHLBI, www.nhlbi.nih.gov).

Chapter 38

Managing Angina

Angina—chest pain or discomfort that occurs when an area of your heart muscle doesn't get enough oxygen-rich blood—is a symptom of an underlying heart problem, usually heart disease. The types of angina are stable, unstable, variant (Prinzmetal), and microvascular. Knowing how the types differ is important because they have different symptoms and require different treatments.

Types of Angina

Stable Angina

Stable angina is the most common type of angina. It occurs if the heart is working harder than usual. Stable angina has a regular pattern. It doesn't come as a surprise, and episodes of pain tend to be alike. It usually lasts a short time (five minutes or less) and is relieved by rest or medicine. It may feel like gas, indigestion, or chest pain that spreads to the arms, back, or other areas.

Physical exertion is the most common trigger of stable angina. Severely narrowed arteries may allow enough blood to reach the heart when the demand for oxygen is low, such as when you're sitting. However, with physical exertion—like walking up a hill or climbing stairs—the heart works harder and needs more oxygen. Other triggers of stable angina include emotional stress, exposure to very hot or cold temperatures, heavy meals, and smoking.

If you know you have stable angina, you can learn to recognize the pattern and predict when the pain will occur. The pain usually goes away a few minutes after you rest or take your angina medicine.

Stable angina isn't a heart attack, but it suggests a heart attack is more likely in the future.

Unstable Angina

Unstable angina doesn't follow a pattern. It can occur with or without physical exertion, and it may not be relieved by rest or medicine. It often occurs at rest, while sleeping at night, or with little physical exertion. It is more severe and lasts longer (as long as 30 minutes) than episodes of stable angina. It may continually get worse.

Blood clots that partly or totally block an artery cause unstable angina. If plaque in an artery ruptures, blood clots may form, creating a larger blockage. A clot may grow large enough to completely block the artery and cause a heart attack.

Blood clots may form, partly dissolve, and later form again. Angina can occur each time a clot blocks an artery.

Unstable angina is very dangerous and requires emergency treatment. This type of angina is a sign a heart attack may happen soon.

Variant (Prinzmetal) Angina

Variant angina is rare. It occurs when the muscles around a coronary artery go into spasm. The spasm causes the walls of the artery to tighten and narrow. Blood flow to the affected portion of the heart slows or stops. Usually the vessel walls will relax after a while, but in severe cases, a heart attack can occur.

Variant angina most often occurs while you're at rest and during the night or early morning hours, usually between midnight and early morning. The pain can be severe.

Variant angina is most common in people who have coronary artery disease. However, it can occur in people who don't have heart disease. Women and smokers are more likely to have variant angina. Other factors that can cause the coronary arteries to spasm include exposure to cold, emotional stress, medicines that tighten or narrow blood vessels, and cocaine use.

Medicine can relieve this type of angina.

Microvascular Angina

Microvascular angina is different from other forms of angina in that the blocked vessels are tiny, even microscopic, blood vessels that branch off the large coronary arteries. People with microvascular angina may have normal coronary angiography because the affected vessels are too small to see. The vessel blockages may be due to cholesterol deposits or spasms.

Microvascular angina is more common in women, and about 70% of cases occur in women around the time of menopause. Microvascular angina can be more severe and last longer than other types of angina; medicine may not relieve it. It may occur with shortness of breath, sleep problems, fatigue, and lack of energy. Often it is first noticed during routine daily activities and times of mental stress.

Managing Angina

Managing angina involves lifestyle changes, medicine, medical procedures, cardiac rehabilitation, and other therapies. The main goals of treatment are to reduce pain, discomfort, and how often it occurs and prevent or lower the risk of heart attack and death by treating the underlying heart condition.

Lifestyle changes and medicine may be the only treatments needed if your symptoms are mild and aren't getting worse. When lifestyle changes and medicine don't control angina, you may need medical procedures or cardiac rehabilitation.

Lifestyle Changes

Making lifestyle changes can help prevent episodes of angina. You can slow down or take rest breaks if physical exertion triggers angina, avoid large meals and rich foods that leave you feeling stuffed if heavy meals trigger angina, and try to avoid situations that make you upset or stressed if emotional stress triggers angina. Learn ways to handle stress that can't be avoided.

Medicine

Nitrates are the medicine most commonly used to treat angina. They relax and widen blood vessels, which allows more blood to flow to the heart while reducing the heart's workload.

Nitroglycerin is the most commonly used nitrate for angina. Nitroglycerin that dissolves under your tongue or between your cheek and gum is used to relieve angina episodes. Nitroglycerin pills and skin patches are used to prevent angina episodes. These forms of nitroglycerin act too slowly to relieve pain during an angina attack.

You also may need other medicines to treat angina. These medicines may include beta blockers, calcium channel blockers, ACE (angiotensin-converting enzyme) inhibitors, oral antiplatelet medicines, and anticoagulants (blood thinners).

People who have stable angina may be advised to get annual flu shots.

Medical Procedures

If lifestyle changes and medicine don't control angina, you may need a medical procedure to treat the underlying heart disease. Both angioplasty and coronary artery bypass grafting (CABG) are commonly used to treat heart disease. You will work with your doctor to decide which treatment is right for you.

Cardiac Rehabilitation

Your doctor may recommend cardiac rehab for angina or after angioplasty, CABG, or a heart attack. Cardiac rehab is a medically supervised program that may help improve the health and well-being of people who have heart problems.

Enhanced External Counterpulsation Therapy

Enhanced external counterpulsation (EECP) therapy is helpful for some people who have angina. Large cuffs, similar to blood pressure cuffs, are put on your legs. The cuffs are inflated and deflated in sync with your heartbeat. EECP therapy improves the flow of oxygen-rich blood to the heart muscle and helps relieve angina. You typically get 35 one-hour treatments over seven weeks.

What You Need to Know

Angina isn't a heart attack, but it does increase your risk of having a heart attack. The risk is even higher if you have unstable angina. For these reasons, it's important that you know the usual pattern of your angina, if you have it regularly, what medicines you take (keep a list) and how to take them, how to control your angina, the limits of your physical activity, and how and when to seek medical attention.

Know the Pattern of Your Angina

Stable angina usually occurs in a pattern. You should know what causes the pain to occur, what angina pain feels like, how long the pain usually lasts, and whether rest or medicine relieves the pain.

After several episodes, you'll learn to recognize when you're having angina. You'll want to pay attention to whether the pattern changes. Pattern changes may include angina that occurs more often, lasts longer, is more severe, occurs without physical exertion, or doesn't go away with rest or medicine.

These changes may be a sign your symptoms are getting worse or becoming unstable. You should seek medical help. Unstable angina suggests you're at high risk for a heart attack very soon.

Know Your Medicines

You should know what medicines you're taking, the purpose of each, how and when to take them, and possible side effects. It's very important that you know exactly when and how to take fast-acting nitroglycerin or other nitrates to relieve chest pain.

Knowing how to correctly store your angina medicines and when to replace them also is important. Your doctor can advise you on this.

If you have side effects from your medicine, let your doctor know. You should never stop taking your medicine without your doctor's approval.

Talk with your doctor if you have any questions or concerns about taking your angina medicine. Tell him or her about any other medicines you're taking. Some medicines can cause serious problems if they're taken with nitrates or other angina medicines.

Controlling Your Angina

After several angina episodes, you'll know the level of activity, stress, and other factors that trigger your angina. By knowing this, you can take steps to prevent or lessen the severity of episodes.

Know what level of physical exertion triggers your angina and try to stop and rest before chest pain starts. For example, if walking up a flight of stairs leads to chest pain, then stop halfway and rest before continuing.

When chest pain occurs during physical exertion, stop and rest or take your angina medicine. The pain should go away in a few minutes. If the pain doesn't go away or lasts longer than usual, call 911 for emergency care.

Anger, arguing, and worrying are examples of emotional stress that can trigger angina episodes. Try to avoid or limit situations that cause these emotions.

Exercise and relaxation can help relieve stress. Alcohol and drug use play a part in causing stress and don't relieve it. If stress is a problem for you, talk with your doctor about getting help for it.

If large meals lead to chest pain, eat smaller meals. Also avoid eating rich foods.

Most people who have stable angina can continue their normal activities. This includes work, hobbies, and sexual relations. However, if you do very strenuous activities or have a stressful job, talk with your doctor.

How and When to Seek Medical Attention

Talk with your doctor about making an emergency action plan. The plan should include making sure you and your family members know the signs and symptoms of a heart attack, how to use aspirin and nitroglycerin when needed, how to access emergency medical services in your community, and the location of the nearest hospital that offers 24-hour emergency heart care.

Be sure to discuss your emergency plan with your family members. Take action quickly if your chest pain becomes severe, lasts longer than a few minutes, or isn't relieved by rest or medicine.

Sometimes, it may be hard to tell the difference between unstable angina and a heart attack. Both are emergency situations, so you should call 911 right away.

Excerpted and adapted from "Angina," National Heart, Lung, and Blood Institute (NHLBI, www.nhlbi.nih.gov), March 2010.

Chapter 39

Erectile Dysfunction in Men with Heart Problems

Many men with heart disease complain of sexual difficulties. Sexual problems may precede a diagnosis of heart disease, but it is also not unusual for them to appear following a heart attack or other major cardiac event.

Sexual dysfunction related to heart disease is frequently the result of vascular damage caused by either the heart problem itself or the medications used to treat it. Due to physical differences in sexual response between men and women, these sexual problems disproportionately affect men. Sexual problems can and do occur in women with heart disease, but they are very rarely the direct result of a vascular problem.

Erection Problems

Erection problems can be a difficult topic to discuss, but if you have problems getting or keeping an erection, you have good reasons to talk with a doctor: erection problems not only interfere with your sex life but can also be a sign of other health problems.

Fear and Sexual Activity

Sexual activity is often safe for low-risk heart patients. The maximum heart rate during usual sexual activity is similar to that during other daily activities, such as walking up one or two flights of stairs. Talk to your doctor to find out whether sexual activity is safe for you.

Erection problems can be a symptom of blocked blood vessels or nerve damage from diabetes. If you don't see your doctor, these problems would go untreated and could harm your body.

Erection problems used to be called impotence. Now the term erectile dysfunction is more common. Sometimes people just use the initials ED.

Erection Triggers

Hormones, blood vessels, nerves, and muscles must all work together to cause an erection. Your brain starts an erection by sending nerve signals to the penis when it senses sexual stimulation. Touch may cause this arousal. Other triggers may be things you see or hear or sexual thoughts or dreams.

These nerve signals cause the muscles in the penis to relax and let blood flow into the spongy tissue in the penis. Blood collects in this tissue like water filling a sponge. The penis becomes larger and firmer, like an inflated balloon. The veins then get shut off to keep blood from flowing out.

After climax or after the sexual arousal has passed, the veins open back up and blood flows back into the body.

Evaluation

Talking about ED can be difficult. When you meet with your doctor, you might use a phrase like "I've been having problems in the bedroom" or "I've been having erection problems." Remember that a healthy sex life is part of a healthy life. Don't feel embarrassed about seeking help. ED is a medical problem, and your doctor treats medical problems every day.

If talking with your doctor doesn't put you at ease, ask for a referral to another doctor. Your doctor may send you to a urologist—a doctor who specializes in sexual and urologic problems.

Your partner may want to come with you to see the doctor. Many doctors say ED is easier to treat when both partners are involved.

To find the cause of your ED, your doctor will take a complete medical history and do a physical exam.

Your doctor will ask general questions about your health as well as specific questions about your erection problems and your relationship with your partner. Bring a list of all the medicines you take, or bring them with you to show your doctor. Tell your doctor about any surgery you have had.

A physical exam can help your doctor find the cause of your ED. As part of the exam, the doctor will examine your testes and penis, take your blood pressure, and check your reflexes. A blood sample will be taken to test for diabetes, cholesterol level, and other conditions that may be associated with ED.

Treating ED

Your doctor can offer a number of treatments for ED. You may want to talk with your partner about which treatment fits you best as a couple. Most people want the simplest treatment possible. You may need to try a number of treatments before you find the one that works best for you.

Lifestyle Changes

For some men, getting more exercise, quitting smoking, losing weight, or cutting back on alcohol may solve erection problems.

Counseling

Even though most cases of ED have a physical cause, counseling can help couples deal with the emotional effects. Some couples find counseling adds to the medical treatment by making their relationship stronger.

Oral Medicines

Since 1998, doctors have been able to prescribe a pill to treat ED. Current brands include Viagra®, Levitra®, and Cialis®. If your health is generally good, your doctor may prescribe one of these drugs. You should not take any of these pills to treat ED if you take any nitrates, a type of heart medicine. All ED pills work by increasing blood flow to the penis. They do not cause automatic erections. Talk with your doctor about when to take the pill. You may need to experiment to find out how quickly the pill takes effect.

You cannot take these medications if you use heart medications called nitrates. These include nitroglycerin, isosorbide dinitrate (Isordil®), and isosorbide mononitrate (Imdur®). The combination can cause a severe, even fatal, drop in blood pressure.

If you develop chest pain, you must not use nitroglycerin if you have used one of these ED pills within a certain time frame. For Viagra and Levitra, this is 24 hours. For Cialis, it is 48 hours. You should make emergency medical personnel aware immediately if you have taken these drugs.

Even if taking a pill solves your erection problem, you should still take care of the other health issues that may have caused your ED.

Use Caution with Prescription Medications

Some prescription medications for sexual dysfunction have life-threatening interactions with nitrates. If you are prescribed medication for sexual dysfunction, make sure your doctor knows about all the other medications you are taking. Ask whether you can safely take nitroglycerin if you develop angina.

Injections

Taking a pill doesn't work for everybody. Many men use medicines that go directly into the penis. Caverject® and Edex® are injected into the shaft of the penis with a needle. MUSE® is a tiny pill inserted into the urethra at the tip of the penis. These medicines usually cause an erection within minutes. These medicines can be very successful, even if other treatments fail.

Vacuum Device

Another way to create an erection is to use a specially designed vacuum tube. The penis is inserted into the tube, which is connected to a pump. As air is pumped out of the tube, blood flows into the penis and makes it larger. A specially designed elastic ring is moved from the end of the tube to the base of the penis to keep the blood from flowing out.

Penile Implant

If other options fail, some men need surgery to treat ED. A surgeon can implant a device that inflates or unbends to create an erection. Implanted devices do not interfere with the way sex feels.

Penile implant operations cannot be reversed. Once a man has a penile implant, he must use the device to have an erection. Talk with your doctor about the pros and cons of having a penile implant.

Excerpted and adapted from "Cardiac Rehabilitation," National Heart, Lung, and Blood Institute (NHLBI, www.nhlbi.nih.gov), August 2009, and "What I Need to Know about Erection Problems," National Kidney and Urologic Diseases Information Clearinghouse, a service of the National Institute of Diabetes and Digestive and Kidney Diseases (NIDDK, www.niddk.nih.gov), June 2009, with supplemental information by David A. Cooke, MD, FACP, July 2010.

Chapter 40

What to Do in an Emergency

For many people, the first symptom of heart disease is a heart attack. This means everyone should know how to identify the symptoms of a heart attack and how to get immediate medical help.

Ideally, treatment should start within one hour of the first symptoms. Recognizing the warning signs and getting help quickly can save your life.

Know the Warning Signs

Not all heart attacks begin with sudden, crushing pain, as is often shown on TV or in the movies. Many heart attacks start slowly with mild pain or discomfort. The most common warning signs are the following:

- You may feel chest discomfort. Most heart attacks involve discomfort in the center of the chest that lasts for more than a few minutes. It may feel like uncomfortable pressure, squeezing, fullness, or pain. The discomfort can be mild or severe, and it may come and go.

- Discomfort in other areas of the upper body, including one or both arms or the back, neck, jaw, or stomach, is another common warning sign.

- You may feel shortness of breath, which may occur with or without chest discomfort.

- Other signs include nausea, light-headedness, or breaking out in a cold sweat.

Get Help Quickly

If you think you or someone else may be having a heart attack, you must act quickly to prevent disability or death and to get the most benefit from current treatments. Wait no more than a few minutes—five at most—before calling 911.

It is important to call 911 because emergency medical personnel can begin treatment even before you get to the hospital. They also have the equipment and training to start your heart beating again if it stops. Calling 911 quickly can save your life.

Even if you're not sure you're having a heart attack, call 911 if your symptoms last up to five minutes. If your symptoms stop completely in less than five minutes, you should still call your doctor right away.

You must also act at once because hospitals have clot-dissolving medicine and other artery-opening treatments that can stop a heart attack if administered quickly. These treatments work best when given within the first hour after a heart attack starts.

When you get to the hospital, don't be afraid to speak up for what you need—or bring someone who can speak up for you. Ask for tests to determine if you are having a heart attack. Commonly given initial tests include an EKG and a cardiac blood test (to check for heart damage). You have the right to be thoroughly examined for a possible heart attack. If you are having a heart attack, you have the right to immediate treatment to help stop the attack.

Delay Can Be Deadly

Most people who have a heart attack wait too long to seek medical help, which can be a fatal mistake. Some delay because they don't understand the symptoms of a heart attack and think what they're feeling is due to another cause. Others put off getting help because they don't want to worry others or cause a scene, especially if their symptoms turn out to be a false alarm. Women are especially likely to delay. A large study of heart attack patients found that, on average, women waited 22 minutes longer than men before going to the hospital.

Don't wait. When you're facing something as serious as a possible heart attack, it's much better to be safe than sorry. Waiting too long can cause permanent disability or death. If you have any symptoms of a possible heart attack that last up to five minutes, call 911 right away.

Plan Ahead

Nobody plans on having a heart attack. But just as many people have a plan in case of fire, it is important to make a plan to deal with a possible heart attack. Taking the following steps can preserve your health—and your life.

- Learn the heart attack warning signs.

- Talk with family and friends about the warning signs and the need to call 911 quickly.

- Talk with your doctor about your risk factors for heart attack and how to reduce them.

- Write out a heart attack survival plan that includes important medical information and keep it handy (see figure 40.1).

- Arrange in advance to have someone else care for your children or other dependents in an emergency.

Heart Attack Survival Plan

Fill out the form below and make several copies. Keep one copy near your home phone, where you can easily see it. Keep another copy at work, and a third copy in your wallet or purse.

Information To Share With Emergency Medical Personnel and Hospital Staff

Medicines you are taking:

_____

_____

_____

_____

_____

Medicines you are allergic to:

_____

_____

_____

_____

_____

How To Contact Your Doctor
If symptoms stop completely in less than 5 minutes, you should still call your doctor right away.

Phone number during office hours:_____

Phone number after office hours:_____

Person To Contact If You Go to the Hospital

Name:_____

Home phone number: _____

Work phone number:_____

Figure 40.1. Use this form to write out your heart attack survival plan.

Cardiopulmonary Resuscitation (CPR)

CPR is performed when the heart has stopped or is not pumping effectively. While CPR only occasionally saves a life by itself, it is critical for allowing time for other life-saving treatment. CPR buys a dying patient time and improves his or her chances of survival.

CPR is relatively simple to learn and perform. Formal CPR classes are offered throughout the United States at many schools, libraries, hospitals, and other organizations. Taking a class is helpful because it allows for hands-on training and practice on a simulated patient mannequin. However, most people can follow instructions for CPR without prior training in an emergency.

The following recommendations are based on the 2005 American Heart Association guidelines on CPR. These guidelines are being updated at press time, so the final 2010 recommendations may differ somewhat from what is presented here. However, the current technique is tried and tested and will improve the odds of survival.

Step 1: Assess Responsiveness

Determine whether the victim is truly unresponsive or merely asleep. Tap the person on the shoulder and ask in a loud voice, "Are you all right?" If the victim does not respond, proceed to the next step of CPR.

Step 2: Activate the EMS System, Call 911

Getting more advanced help is critical for the victim's survival. If you are alone, call 911 immediately, even if this means leaving the victim. If emergency medical services (EMS) are not called promptly, the chances of survival will be very slim. If an automated external defibrillator (AED) is available, get the AED after calling 911, then return to the victim.

If more than one person is present, send someone else to call 911 and get the AED (if one is available).

Step 3: Open the Airway and Check Breathing

Once EMS has been called, roll the victim onto his or her back. A hard surface such as a floor is best; it is very difficult to perform CPR on a bed or other soft surface.

Place one hand on the victim's forehead and the other hand on his or her jaw. Tilt the head backward and lift the jaw to open the mouth. Leave the head and neck in this position.

Place your ear a few inches above the victim's mouth and look at his or her chest. Look for rising and falling of the chest. Listen for sounds of breathing from the mouth. Feel for the victim's breath on your face.

If the victim is breathing, keep him or her in this position and watch to ensure the victim keeps breathing until EMS arrives.

If you cannot see, hear, or feel breathing within 10 seconds, proceed to the next step of CPR.

Step 4: Give Rescue Breaths

If the victim is not breathing, keep his or her head tilted back, pinch the victim's nose shut with your fingers, and seal your lips over his or her mouth. This is known as mouth-to-mouth resuscitation. Blow into the victim's mouth with a regular breath over one second, just enough to make the chest rise. Break the seal, and let the victim exhale.

Give a second breath within a few seconds of the first, using the same technique.

If you attempt to give a breath and it does not go in, the airway is not open. Tilt the head back again and open the mouth. Try to give another breath. If it still does not go in, reposition again and repeat.

Some rescuers do not feel comfortable giving mouth-to-mouth resuscitation, particularly to a stranger. CPR without mouth-to-mouth resuscitation may be less effective than with it, but it is clearly superior to no CPR at all. If you cannot give mouth-to-mouth resuscitation, proceed with CPR without providing breaths.

Step 5: Chest Compressions

If the victim is not breathing, it is likely his or her heart has stopped as well. Chest compressions will help circulate blood to the vital organs while waiting for EMS to arrive.

If an AED is available, turn it on and attach it to the victim. Follow the prompts from the AED.

If an AED is not available, or if it does not recommend a shock, start chest compressions. Kneel at the victim's side and put the heel of one hand in the center of the chest, between the nipples. Place your other hand over the first one so the heel of one hand is covering the other.

Press down hard on the victim's chest so that the chest moves down about 1½–2 inches. Release and let the chest spring back before starting the next compression.

Repeat compressions, aiming for about 100 per minute. Each compression should take a bit more than half a second. CPR is most effective when it is done fast and hard!

Perform 30 compressions, then pause and give an additional two breaths by mouth-to-mouth resuscitation.

Resume compressions, and repeat at a ratio of 30 cycles to two breaths. Do not stop to check a pulse or for breathing.

Continue the compression/breathing cycles until an AED is available, EMS arrives, or you are too tired to continue.

If more than one rescuer is available, switching off every two minutes (or five cycles of 30 compression and two breaths) will help prevent exhaustion.

Other Considerations about CPR

It is common to hear or feel ribs break during CPR. This is not a reason to stop. Better to live with broken ribs than to die with them intact!

It is important to understand that even with expert CPR and prompt EMS arrival, survival rates after CPR tend to be poor. This does not mean you failed or performed CPR incorrectly. Most cardiac arrest victims do not recover, despite rescuers' best efforts.

Even so, if only a small fraction of people who receive CPR live, this still amounts to many lives saved each year. Survival is much better with CPR than without CPR, and clumsy CPR is much better than no CPR at all!

Where to Learn CPR

Many organizations offer CPR training, and classes are likely offered in your area. Schools, hospitals, houses of worship, and service organizations frequently sponsor classes. Some organizations offer courses for free and others for a nominal charge. The following resources may be helpful in locating classes:

American Heart Association
The American Heart Association issues standards and guidelines for CPR and offers classes and CPR instructor certification. Information can be obtained by telephone by calling 800-AHA-USA-1 or 800-242-8721. An online class locator can also be accessed from the American Heart Association website at: www.americanheart.org.

American Red Cross
The American Red Cross offers classes in first aid, CPR, and AED use. Information on local classes is best obtained by contacting your local American Red Cross chapter. If you have difficulty locating your local chapter, the American Red Cross national telephone number is 202-303-5000. An online class locator can also be accessed from the American Red Cross website at www.redcross.org.

Automated External Defibrillators

An AED is a portable device that checks the heart rhythm and can send an electric shock to the heart to try to restore a normal rhythm. AEDs are used to treat sudden cardiac arrest (SCA).

SCA usually causes death if it's not treated within minutes. In fact, each minute of SCA leads to a 10% reduction in survival. Using an AED on a person who is having SCA may save the person's life.

Ninety-five percent of people who have SCA die from it—most within minutes. Rapid treatment of SCA with an AED can be life-saving.

When to Use an AED

The most common cause of SCA is an arrhythmia called ventricular fibrillation (v-fib). In v-fib, the ventricles (the heart's lower chambers) don't beat normally. Instead, they quiver very rapidly and irregularly.

Another arrhythmia that can lead to SCA is ventricular tachycardia, a fast, regular beating of the ventricles that may last for a few seconds or much longer.

In people who have either of these arrhythmias, an electric shock from an AED can restore the heart's normal rhythm (if done within minutes of the onset of SCA).

If someone is having SCA, you may see him or her suddenly collapse and lose consciousness. Or you may find the person unconscious and unable to respond when you call or shake him or her.

The person may not be breathing, or he or she may have an abnormal breathing pattern. If you check, you usually can't find a pulse. The person's skin also may become dark or blue from lack of oxygen. Also, the person may not move, or his or her movements may look like a seizure (spasms).

An AED can check the person's heart rhythm and determine whether an electric shock is needed to try to restore a normal rhythm.

How AEDs Work

Automated external defibrillators are lightweight, battery-operated, portable devices that are easy to use. Sticky pads with sensors (called electrodes) are attached to the chest of the person who is having SCA.

The electrodes transmit information about the person's heart rhythm to a computer in the AED. The computer analyzes the heart rhythm to find out whether an electric shock is needed. If a shock is needed, the AED uses voice prompts to tell you when to give the shock, and the electrodes deliver it.

Using an AED to shock the heart within minutes of the start of SCA may restore a normal heart rhythm.

Training

Learning how to use an AED and taking a CPR course are helpful. However, if trained personnel aren't available, untrained people also can use an AED to help save someone's life.

Some people are afraid to use an AED to help save someone's life. They're worried that something might go wrong and that they might be sued. However, Good Samaritan laws in each state and the Federal Cardiac Arrest Survival Act (CASA) provide some protection for untrained bystanders who respond to emergencies.

Facility owners who are thinking about buying an AED should provide initial and ongoing training to likely rescuers (usually people who work in the facility). Also, it's important to properly maintain an AED and notify local emergency officials of its location.

Before Using an AED

Before using an automated external defibrillator on someone you think is having sudden cardiac arrest, it's important to check him or her.

If you see a person suddenly collapse and lose consciousness, or if you find a person already unconscious, confirm that the person can't respond. Shout at and shake the person to make sure he or she isn't sleeping.

Never shake an infant or young child. Instead, pinch the child to try to wake him or her up.

Call 911 or have someone else call 911. If two rescuers are present, one can provide CPR while the other calls 911 and gets the AED.

Check the person's breathing and pulse. If breathing and pulse are absent or irregular, prepare to use the AED as soon as possible.

If no one knows how long the person has been unconscious, or if an AED isn't readily available, do two minutes of CPR. Then use the AED (if you have one) to check the person.

After you use the AED, or if you don't have an AED, give CPR until emergency medical help arrives or until the person begins to move. Try to limit pauses in CPR. After two minutes of CPR, you can use the AED again to check the person's heart rhythm and give another shock, if needed. If a shock isn't needed, continue CPR.

Using an AED

AEDs are user-friendly devices that untrained bystanders can use to save the life of someone having SCA.

Before using an AED, check for puddles or water near the person who is unconscious. Move him or her to a dry area and stay away from wetness when delivering shocks (water conducts electricity).

Turn on the AED's power. The device will give you step-by-step instructions. You'll hear voice prompts and see prompts on a screen.

Expose the person's chest. If the person's chest is wet, dry it. AEDs have sticky pads with sensors called electrodes. Apply the pads to the person's chest as pictured on the AED's instructions.

Place one pad on the right center of the person's chest above the nipple. Place the other pad slightly below the other nipple and to the left on the rib cage.

Make sure the sticky pads have good connection with the skin. If the connection isn't good, the machine may repeat the phrase "check electrodes."

If the person has a lot of chest hair, you may have to trim it. (AEDs usually come with a kit that includes scissors and/or a razor.) If the person is wearing a medication patch that's in the way, remove it and clean the medicine from the skin before applying the sticky pads.

Remove metal necklaces and underwire bras. The metal may conduct electricity and cause burns. You can cut the center of the bra and pull it away from the skin.

Check the person for implanted medical devices, such as pacemakers or implantable cardioverter defibrillators. (The outline of these devices is visible under the skin on the chest or abdomen, and the person may be wearing a medical alert bracelet.) Also check for body piercings.

Move the defibrillator pads at least one inch away from implanted devices or piercings so the electric current can flow freely between the pads.

Check that the wires from the electrodes are connected to the AED. Make sure no one is touching the person, and then press the AED's "analyze" button. Stay clear while the machine checks the person's heart rhythm.

If a shock is needed, the AED will let you know when to deliver it. Stand clear of the person and make sure others are clear before you push the AED's "shock" button.

Start or resume CPR until emergency medical help arrives or until the person begins to move. Stay with the person until medical help arrives, and report all the information you know about what has happened.

Risks

Automated external defibrillators are safe to use. There are no reports of AEDs harming bystanders or users. Also, there are no reports of AEDs delivering inappropriate shocks.

If someone is having SCA, using an AED and giving CPR can improve the person's chance of survival.

Excerpted and adapted from "Your Guide to Living Well with Heart Disease," November 2005, with facts about AEDs excerpted from "Automated External Defibrillator," December 2009, both produced by the National Heart, Lung, and Blood Institute (NHLBI, www.nhlbi.nih.gov), with supplemental information about CPR written by David A. Cooke, MD, FACP, April 2010.

Part Four

Research and Resources

Many people with heart disease have questions about medical research and how the results of current studies may alter our understanding of heart disease or lead to innovative treatments. This last part of the book begins with information about current research initiatives.

One area of particular interest is the role of inflammation as a risk factor for heart disease or the recurrence of heart problems. Although inflammation is part of the body's normal process of healing, researchers have discovered it can also lead to the development of atherosclerosis. A particular protein that develops in the body in response to inflammation, C-reactive protein, may serve to help physicians better understand which patients face an elevated risk of heart attack. A chapter about inflammation explains why treating underlying inflammation may become an important strategy in the battle against heart disease.

The next chapter discusses a number of other studies that have pointed to a relationship between air pollution and heart disease. Although it may not be practical for people to move out of urban areas, an understanding of how air quality may impact heart health can help patients take appropriate precautions when the Air Quality Index indicates unhealthy or hazardous conditions.

Another area of recent research has focused on what has become known as the metabolic syndrome—a common clustering of symptoms linked with the development of heart disease. Although much remains unknown, including whether or not these symptoms result from an underlying common cause, a chapter about current discoveries reveals that addressing the individual components may help modify a person's ultimate risk for heart-related problems or their recurrence.

In addition, some people with heart disease wonder whether chelation treatments that claim to clear blocked arteries actually work. A chapter about chelation therapy reviews what researchers have discovered and discusses the risks associated with the chemicals most frequently used.

After addressing these topics, this part turns its focus to identifying resources that can help you find additional information. Because nutrition often plays an important role in recovery, a chapter on finding heart-healthy recipes lists cookbooks and websites to help you keep mealtimes tasty and satisfying. It also includes a few sample recipes you can try right away. Finally, an annotated resource directory includes details about many organizations that are able to help you better understand your own heart condition and support you in your journey back to wellness.

Chapter 41

The Metabolic Syndrome

The metabolic syndrome, also known as metabolic syndrome X, was first described in 1988. It was recognized as a common clustering of clinical symptoms strongly associated with cardiovascular disease. Over the past two decades, there has been considerable research and study of the metabolic syndrome, and some of its elements are now better understood. Nevertheless, many unknowns remain, and experts continue to debate whether the metabolic syndrome is a distinct disease or a combination of several different disorders.

Defining the Metabolic Syndrome
Several definitions of the metabolic syndrome have been issued since it was first described. However, they were considered unsatisfactory because they required complex testing to make the diagnosis. The 2005 American Heart Association/National Heart, Blood, and Lung Institute definition is simpler and based on common tests, and it is now the most widely used standard. Under this

definition, a person is said to have the metabolic syndrome if at least three of five elements are present:

- Waist circumference greater than 40 inches in men or 35 inches in women; a smaller standard, 35 inches in men or 31 inches in women, is recommended for Asian Americans

- Fasting triglycerides greater than 150 mg/dl (milligrams per deciliter); or on medication for elevated triglycerides

- HDL cholesterol less than 40 mg/dl in men or 50 mg/dl in women; or on medication for low HDL cholesterol

- Systolic blood pressure greater than 130 mmHg (millimeters of mercury) or diastolic blood pressure greater than 85 mmHg; or on medication for elevated blood pressure

- Fasting glucose >100 mg/dl; or on medication for elevated glucose

In the United States, it is estimated that about 25% of people aged 25–59 meet this definition of the metabolic syndrome, and more than 40% of people older than 60 have the condition.

The fact that these particular elements are so frequently seen together has led many researchers to suspect they are all manifestations of a single underlying disease. However, this point remains very controversial, and research to date has not provided a clear answer.

Causes of the Metabolic Syndrome

Obesity is believed to play a critical role in the metabolic syndrome. Rates of obesity have been rapidly increasing in the United States in recent decades, and high rates of the metabolic syndrome are directly linked to obesity. While obesity is not required for a diagnosis of the metabolic syndrome, nearly all people with the metabolic syndrome are obese.

Excess fat is believed to be the root cause of the metabolic syndrome. Most people think of fat as inert tissue. In fact, fat tissue is very hormonally active and constitutes a major endocrine organ in the human body.

Fat can be stored in a number of locations in the body, including the trunk, hips, legs, and surrounding the abdominal organs. Its location in a given person is determined by genetic, hormonal, and gender-specific factors. Research suggests the location of a person's fat has more than cosmetic significance.

Not all fat seems to be the same. Fat deposits around the abdominal organs, known as visceral fat, behave somewhat differently than other fat. Abdominal obesity typically reflects increased amounts of visceral fat, which is why waist circumference is considered in the definition of metabolic syndrome

Visceral fat is located next to the abdominal organs, so hormones from visceral fat release into the blood and drain directly into the liver. The liver has a central role in metabolism, which amplifies the effects of the fat hormones. These interactions trigger a complex cascade of metabolic changes that lead to elevated levels of blood fats, low levels of HDL cholesterol, resistance to the effects of insulin, and increases in blood pressure.

These hormonal effects also appear to interact with the immune system. The metabolic syndrome promotes inflammation, which appears critical to the development of atherosclerosis. Markers of inflammation are frequently elevated in the blood of people with the metabolic syndrome, and high levels are known to predict cardiovascular disease. Additionally, active inflammation promotes blood clotting, which is often the inciting event in a heart attack or stroke.

Excess visceral fat appears to be necessary for the metabolic syndrome to develop, but it may not be enough by itself. It is believed that a number of genetic variations affect the risk for the metabolic syndrome and that the condition is at least partially hereditary. Not all obese individuals develop the metabolic syndrome, and some people show symptoms of the metabolic syndrome with much less obesity than others.

There are definite racial differences in the frequency of the metabolic syndrome, which cannot simply be explained by differences in rates of obesity. The metabolic syndrome is more common in white men than African American men, and people of Mexican, Native American, and Pacific Islander descent seem to have higher risk than whites. Many people of Asian descent develop the abnormalities of the metabolic syndrome with only mild obesity, which is why a smaller waist circumference is used in the clinical definition. Studies have also shown increased risk for the metabolic syndrome within individual families.

It has been speculated that the genes that predispose a person to the metabolic syndrome may reflect adaptations that were useful over most of human history. Some of these metabolic changes allow for more efficient metabolism when food is scarce and may reduce the risk of starvation. However, under conditions where food is plentiful, their effects are more harmful.

Dietary factors are also important. The metabolic syndrome is much more common among people who follow Western-style diets and is more common in cities than in rural areas.

Finally, lack of exercise also appears to be a major contributing factor. Poor physical fitness and little leisure-time physical activity are strongly correlated with the metabolic syndrome.

The Significance of the Metabolic Syndrome

The metabolic syndrome is critical in that it strongly predicts cardiovascular disease. People with the metabolic syndrome were 1.5 to 2.7 times more likely to have heart attacks or strokes in several large population studies. The risk of developing diabetes is approximately three times the average. Other studies have found the overall risk of death for people with the metabolic syndrome to be 37–60% higher than for people without it. Given how many people have the metabolic syndrome, this may translate into millions of deaths and billions of dollars in medical costs each year.

The metabolic syndrome is also strongly associated with fatty liver disease, polycystic ovary syndrome, gout, and sleep apnea. There should be a higher suspicion for these disorders if the metabolic syndrome is present.

Despite these associations and a workable definition, there is still disagreement over whether the metabolic syndrome is actually a disease versus a collection of different conditions. It was originally believed insulin resistance was the root cause of the metabolic syndrome, but it appears the metabolic syndrome can exist in its absence. Some experts argue that the metabolic syndrome is a single disorder with several different effects. Others argue it is not really a condition but simply the presence of several individual cardiac risk factors.

The data so far have not been conclusive. Some studies have found that people with the metabolic syndrome have a higher risk of cardiovascular disease than would be expected from their individual diseases. However, other studies have concluded that the cardiovascular risks seen with the metabolic syndrome are no higher than the risks of the individual diseases present. Indeed, several studies have found that making a diagnosis of the metabolic syndrome predicts risk no better than other assessment methods. Experts continue to disagree over whether the metabolic syndrome is more than the sum of its parts.

Treatment of the Metabolic Syndrome

Whether or not the metabolic syndrome has a special effect on risk, it is clear that people with the condition are in danger of developing cardiovascular disease. There is broad agreement that modifiable risk factors should be treated.

Weight loss is probably the most important and effective measure for treating the metabolic syndrome. Losing 7 to 10% of initial body weight over 6 to 12 months sharply improves the abnormalities of the metabolic syndrome. One study found a 41% reduction in the incidence of the metabolic syndrome, and another found a 58% reduction in the development of diabetes, with weight loss and lifestyle changes. Studies of patients who have undergone weight loss surgery have found dramatic reductions in the rate of the metabolic syndrome.

Increasing exercise is closely tied to weight loss and improvement in the metabolic syndrome. Increased exercise causes hormonal signaling that offsets many of the metabolic syndrome changes and improves insulin resistance. Most experts recommend physical activity of 30–60 minutes daily.

Dietary change is also important in achieving weight loss and treating the metabolic syndrome. It is controversial whether any particular diet is superior for treating the metabolic syndrome, but reducing caloric intake is clearly necessary. Many experts recommend a low-fat diet, with no more than 25% to 35% of daily calories from fat and no more than 7% from saturated fats. Increased intake of fruits, vegetables, and whole grains is also commonly recommended.

Treatment of hypertension is important. Blood pressure should be reduced to no more than 140/90 mmHg, and the American Diabetes Association recommends less than 130/80 mmHg for people with diabetes or kidney disease. If this cannot be achieved through weight loss, diet, and exercise, medication should be used to help reach these targets.

Improving cholesterol levels is a major goal. The recommendations for diabetics are LDL cholesterol less than 100 mg/dl, triglycerides less than 150 mg/dl, and HDL cholesterol greater than 40 mg/dl in men and 50 mg/dl in women. Some authorities recommend the same cholesterol targets for people with the metabolic syndrome, even if they do not have diabetes. Statin medications for high cholesterol are known to reduce the risk of and have beneficial effects on heart disease. Fibrate medications, niacin, and fish oil may also be beneficial, but evidence supporting these is much weaker.

Tight blood sugar control for diabetics with the metabolic syndrome is strongly recommended. As with blood pressure and cholesterol, it is preferable to achieve this through lifestyle changes, but medication should be used if necessary.

It has been suggested that certain medications for diabetes, such as metformin, rosiglitazone, and pioglitazone, may be particularly useful in treating the metabolic syndrome. These medications reduce insulin resistance, and rosiglitazone and pioglitazone appear to reduce visceral fat deposits. However, their benefit over other medications for treating the metabolic syndrome has not been proven. In trials of these medications in people who have the metabolic syndrome without diabetes, the benefits have not been large enough to recommend routine use.

Addressing other cardiovascular risk factors is also important. Smoking cessation is critical, as smoking sharply increases cardiovascular risk when combined with the metabolic syndrome. Low-dose daily aspirin therapy may be recommended for some people given that it reduces risk of heart attack and stroke in high-risk individuals.

If the metabolic syndrome is truly a distinct disorder, it is possible a medication could be developed to treat the core abnormality. In theory, this could treat several individual diseases at the same time. However, researchers have not yet found a single root cause for the disorder.

Conclusion

The metabolic syndrome is very common in the United States, and rates are increasing. It carries a high risk for developing diabetes, heart attack, and stroke. The sheer number of people affected by the condition means many people suffer disability or death from its complications, and the costs of treating the disease are enormous.

Researchers continue to look for additional interventions to address the underlying causes of the disease. It is possible a drug for treating the metabolic syndrome as a whole will eventually be developed.

Until that time, weight loss, dietary change, and increased exercise are clearly effective treatments for the metabolic syndrome and can lead to a cure if they are maintained. Addressing modifiable risk factors such as high blood pressure, high cholesterol, elevated blood sugars, and smoking reduces the risk of bad outcomes.

By David A. Cooke, MD, FACP, April 2010.

Chapter 42

Inflammation as a Risk for Coronary Heart Disease

Inflammation is a process the body uses to heal itself when tissues have been injured or infected. Although it is generally a beneficial process, inflammation may also play a role in the development of coronary atherosclerosis.

Certain risk factors for coronary artery disease have been recognized for some time, including high cholesterol, high blood pressure, tobacco use, sedentary lifestyle, diabetes, male gender, increased age, and family history of heart attack. Some of these risk factors can be changed by diet, exercise, and medication. However, some people continue to have heart problems despite management of their traditional risk factors.

Recently, inflammation has been determined to be a risk factor for atherosclerosis. Inflammation and its associated chemical processes appear to increase a person's risk for disability or death from coronary artery disease. The effects of inflammation appear to add to the effects of other risk factors.

Low-Grade Inflammation

The idea that chronic infection can lead to other disease is already well accepted by doctors. For example, infection with the bacterium *Helicobacter pylori* is a major cause of stomach ulcers. Therefore, some ulcers may be permanently cured with antibiotic treatment. Similarly, scientists have suspected that bacteria or viruses may cause or aggravate atherosclerosis. For example, research has suggested that either the bacterium *Chlamydia pneumoniae* or the herpes simplex virus may be associated with atherosclerotic plaque. However, it remains unclear whether these infections actually cause the disease. In fact, trials of antibiotics have failed to show an effect on atherosclerotic disease.

What has been determined is that the more traditional causes of atherosclerosis cause inflammation. Cigarette smoking, high blood pressure, high cholesterol, and high blood sugar all injure blood vessel walls. When the vessels are damaged, they release inflammatory chemicals. These chemicals attract and change the behavior of white blood cells. This chain of events appears to contribute to the formation of plaque in the coronary arteries. If the plaque then deteriorates, it can cause a heart attack. Each stage in the cascade of events in the development of atherosclerosis involves substances or cells involved in a low-grade inflammatory response.

C-reactive protein and Heart Disease

When inflammation is present in the body, a protein called C-reactive protein (CRP) is produced by the immune system and distributed throughout the body via the circulatory system. Because the amount of CRP in the blood rises as inflammation worsens, a test that measures the level of CRP has been developed to diagnose or monitor some kinds of infections. An improved version of this CRP test, the high-sensitivity CRP (hs-CRP) test, is now coming into widespread use. Among patients who have already had a heart attack, the hs-CRP may be used to gauge the risk of a so-called recurrent coronary event, such as a fatal or nonfatal heart attack or sudden death due to heart dysfunction.

CRP Testing and Risk Assessment of Subsequent Cardiovascular Events

In people who have already had a heart attack, elevated levels of hs-CRP consistently predict the recurrence of heart-related problems. Among patients who have undergone balloon angioplasty to reopen a blocked artery, high levels of hs-CRP in the blood suggest an increased risk for having the affected artery re-close with a clot. Similarly, high levels of hs-CRP suggest patients with stroke or peripheral arterial disease will experience a recurrence.

Elevated hs-CRP levels also suggest patients are less likely to survive another cardiac event. Currently, most authorities believe the hs-CRP assay is a useful tool for predicting the risk a heart patient will have heart problems again.

First-Time Cardiovascular Events and hs-CRP Levels

At one time, researchers wondered if hs-CRP could also identify heart-related risks in people who had not already suffered a heart attack. Studies that followed groups of people over time and that included men, women, and the elderly suggested the higher the hs-CRP level, the greater the risk of having a heart attack. In particular, the risk for heart attack in individuals in the highest third of hs-CRP levels appears to be twice the risk of those with an hs-CRP level in the lower third.

Although there is some evidence of an association between sudden cardiac death, peripheral arterial disease, and hs-CRP, more research is necessary to determine the exact association between hs-CRP and new cardiovascular problems. Some studies have reported hs-CRP improves the prediction of heart disease, but others found the information adds very little.

Should You Have Your CRP Level Measured?

You can discuss with your doctor whether or not you should have your CRP level tested. You doctor can help you understand your cardiovascular risk score, a way to calculate risk based on modifiable and nonmodifiable factors. In general, if your cardiovascular risk score is low (for example, if your risk factors suggest the possibility you will develop cardiovascular disease is less than 10% in 10 years), a CRP test is not indicated. The American Heart Association recommends CRP testing if your cardiovascular risk score is in the intermediate range (for example, between 10% and 20% over the next 10 years) because CRP levels can help guide the need for further evaluation and possible therapy. Individuals with a high risk score, for example (greater than 20% in 10 years), or those who already have heart disease probably do not need CRP testing. That's because they are candidates for aggressive treatment regardless of their hs-CRP level.

Range of hs-CRP Levels

The following hs-CRP levels indicate different levels of risk:

- Below 1 mg/L (milligram per liter) indicates a low risk of developing cardiovascular disease.

- Between 1 and 3 mg/L indicates an average risk.

- Higher than 3 mg/L indicates high risk.

If your hs-CRP is elevated, the test usually should be repeated after several weeks to months. Issues unrelated to cardiac risk, such as a recent illness, can temporarily elevate CRP levels Patients with persistently unexplained and very high hs-CRP (greater than 10 mg/L) should be evaluated for other causes of the elevation because very elevated CRP levels are sometimes a sign of undetected cancer, autoimmune diseases, or other infectious diseases.

Mechanisms by which CRP Raises Coronary Risk

Why increased CRP levels are linked to increased risks for heart problems remains unclear. In fact, scientists are not sure CRP itself is responsible for increased heart disease risk. Instead, elevated

CRP may simply be an indicator of other factors that actually cause damage. However, some researchers believe CRP itself may be responsible.

One theory is that CRP may interfere with the ability of the inner lining of the arteries to respond to calls for changes in blood flow or pressure. If you have coronary artery disease, this development is not a good sign.

On the other hand, CRP may directly promote the formation and progression of atherosclerosis through a number of other means. One possible direct effect involves the way CRP enhances the formation of foam cells. Foam cells are groups of white blood cells that consume foreign material as well as muscle cells in blood vessels that have taken up particles composed of fat-protein from the blood. Foam cells in themselves do not pose a great risk for a coronary event. But a large accumulation of these bloated cells can be troubling if the fibrous cap in the artery wall that covers them breaks into the main passage of a coronary artery.

This development can cause the formation of a blood clot that could block the flow of blood to a portion of the heart muscle. This blockage starves the muscle of oxygen, which is called ischemia. Ischemia can kill the heart muscle, which causes ineffective heart rhythms and contractions—and possibly even death.

Another direct method by which CRP could promote atherosclerosis includes the recruitment of monocytes (another type of white cell) into the arterial wall. This stimulates the development of factors in the tissue that promote clot formation.

Other Conditions Associated with Inflammation and Coronary Artery Disease

Air Pollution and Risk of Coronary Artery Disease

Some forms of air pollution, especially particulate pollution (tiny particles in the air), can suddenly increase the risk of blood clots, which may lead to an increased risk of heart attacks, angina, or dangerously irregular heart rhythms. Collectively, these problems are referred to as ischemic events.

Researchers are undecided how particulate pollution could trigger these ischemic events. It may be that breathing toxic particulate matter can cause inflammation in parts of the lung, which could then lead to worsening pre-existing lung disease and increasing the tendency of blood to coagulate. Such heightened blood coagulability is a setup for premature clotting of an inflamed, narrowed section of coronary artery. Several recent studies of controlled exposures to particulate matter pollution seem to support this hypothesis.

HIV/AIDs

Low-level chronic HIV infection promotes persistent immune activation and inflammation, which may explain why people with HIV are at higher risk for cardiovascular disease, even when their immune functions remain adequate. The usefulness of CRP as a predictor of heart disease in patients with chronic inflammatory conditions such as HIV infection is not clear. Still, it is interesting to speculate that a CRP test might prove useful in assessing cardiovascular risk in patients with other types of inflammation.

Psoriasis

Although psoriasis primarily affects the skin, it is a systemic, immune-mediated disease that often affects other tissues. The association between psoriasis and cardiovascular disease is significant: a 30-year-old patient with severe psoriasis has three times the risk of having a heart attack than a person of the same age without psoriasis.

Systemic Lupus Erythematosus

Systemic lupus erythematosus (SLE) involves inflammation in the connective tissue of many tissues and organs, including blood vessels, skin, joints, muscles, kidneys, lungs, and the central nervous system. SLE, which affects women nine times more often than men, is associated with several cardiovascular problems. In patients with SLE, early atherosclerosis with coronary heart disease is a significant cause of sickness and premature death.

Rheumatoid Arthritis

Rheumatoid arthritis (RA), like psoriasis and systemic lupus erythematosus, is an immune-mediated disease. The disorder involves inflammation of the lubricating tissues inside joints, associated destructive joint changes, and potentially severe disability.

Patients with RA are known to have a 1½- to 2-fold increased risk for blood vessel problems. Although patients with RA tend to have fewer instances of angina (chest pain due to oxygen-starved heart muscle), they are subject to a higher incidence of sudden death and undetected blockages in the heart. The inflammation associated with RA appears to play a role in this excess risk. Anti-rheumatic drugs reduce vascular risk, but chronic high-dose steroids may aggravate vascular risk.

Patients with RA should undergo screening to determine their risk for developing cardiovascular disease. Doctors of patients with high risk may prescribe statin medications. Doctors of patients with other cardiovascular risk factors in addition to RA—such as hypertension, obesity, smoking, and diabetes—may want to take additional steps to help prevent the development of heart disease.

Treatment of High CRP

The treatment of inflammation signaled by high CRP may involve lifestyle changes, including weight loss, increased exercise, management of diabetes, smoking cessation, stabilization of high blood pressure, and reduction of alcohol intake. The physician may prescribe anticlotting medications such as aspirin or clopidogrel. He or she may also prescribe cholesterol-lowering statin drugs and ACE inhibitors to reduce inflammation and lower CRP.

Data from the large JUPITER (Justification for the Use of Statins in Primary Prevention) trial, published in the *New England Journal of Medicine* in 2008, revealed that the drug rosuvastatin (a cholesterol-lowering statin drug) reduced the risk of future serious cardiovascular events in patients with elevated CRP even if their cholesterol levels were normal. It appears that all statin drugs lower CRP, but other drugs have not been well studied in patients whose major cardiac risk is elevated CRP.

Summary

Accumulating evidence in recent years suggests that inflammation plays a key role in coronary artery disease. Too much inflammation, as occurs with chronic infection, rheumatoid arthritis, psoriasis, systemic lupus erythematosus, and perhaps with being overweight or having high cholesterol, appears to facilitate damage to the delicate lining of artery walls and promote the formation and rupture of fatty plaques.

Although no one knows exactly how many people suffer from excess inflammation, physicians can detect it by testing for CRP. Inflammation as evidenced by elevated CRP levels may indicate a need for further evaluation to consider the possible presence of an undetected disorder, the need for lifestyle changes, or the potential benefits of medication.

By Daniel Hayes, MD, April 2010.

Chapter 43

Air Pollution and Heart Disease

Air pollution has become a major problem in modern society. It contributes significantly to illnesses and deaths related to heart disease according to a number of studies conducted over the past 15 years among large populations of people. This increased risk comes in the form of both short- and long-term exposure to air pollution, especially particulate matter.

The goal of this chapter is to help you understand the relationship between air pollution and cardiovascular disease. It begins by discussing how air pollutants are classified, the most common elements in air pollution, and common sources of air pollution. The remaining sections discuss select pollutants in greater detail and what is known about their effects on certain types of heart disease.

Classification of Air Pollutants

Air pollutants may be classified as gases, liquids, or solids. Solids usually occur in the form of tiny particles (particulate matter). However, air pollution rarely contains just one of these forms of pollutants.

The Contents of Polluted Air

In reality, the air you breathe is often polluted by a complex mixture of gases, liquids, and particulate matter. Although air pollution is usually the most intense in dense urban and industrial areas, virtually every spot on the globe is affected.

Specific substances contained in air pollution include smoke, carbon monoxide, carbon dioxide, ozone, oxides of nitrogen, sulfur dioxide, lead, secondhand tobacco smoke, and particulate matter. Some elements of air pollution are from natural sources and others are from human sources.

Examples of Natural Sources

- Forest fires create particulate matter, gases, and volatile organic compounds (substances that take the form of gases in atmosphere).

- Weather and water lead to soil erosion and ultrafine dust.

- Volcanoes are a source of sulfur dioxide and large amounts of volcanic ash.

- Vegetation releases carbon dioxide, pollens, and mold spores.

Human Sources of Air Pollutants

Many pollutants are released into the air as a result of human activity. The most commonly recognized man-made air pollution is smog, which is caused by sunlight interacting with exhaust from motor vehicles and factories.

Other human sources of particulate matter include deteriorating tires, road dust, the by-products of generating power, industrial combustion, metal processing, construction or demolition, and burning.

As you would expect, the concentration of pollutants in the air is greatest in dense urban or industrial areas.

Specific Substances in Air Pollution

Particulate Matter

Particulate matter is made up of both solid and liquid particles. Such particles include nitrates, sulfates, carbon compounds, metals, organic compounds, biological compounds (such as cell fragments), and metals.

The adverse effects of particulate matter on heart function have been known for some time. In 1994, the *Annual Reviews of Public Health* published data from a study showing that for each 10-milligram increase in particulate matter per cubic meter of air, the rate of death from cardiovascular causes increased 1.4%. Hospital admissions for heart failure and coronary artery disease also go up when the presence of particulate matter increases.

Researchers have found evidence that the increased risk of sudden death with exposure to particulate matter may be related to a sudden increase in heart rate or blood pressure or a decrease in the ability of the heart to change its rate of beating in response to stress. Also, particulate matter may promote more rapid blood clotting, narrowing arteries, or inflammation.

Nitrogen Dioxide and Other Nitrogen Oxides

Nitrogen oxides are toxic combinations of nitrogen and oxygen. They are dangerous because of how they react with other substances. The most notable nitrogen oxides in the air you breathe are nitric oxide (NO) and nitrogen dioxide (NO_2).

Most nitrogen oxides in outdoor air come from emissions from vehicles and power plants and other sites that burn fossil fuels such as coal. However, nitric oxide and nitrogen dioxide are also released by natural causes such as fires, volcanoes, lightning, and biological processes whereby bacteria assist in the decomposition of a material that contained nitrogen.

Nitrogen dioxide has received a lot of attention and is regulated worldwide. It contributes to the formation of ozone, another element in air pollution.

Nitrogen dioxide levels vary with traffic density and proximity to industrial sources. The indoor concentration of nitrogen dioxide is often higher than the outdoor concentration, especially when gas stoves and kerosene heaters are being used.

Commuters inside vehicles traveling in dense traffic may be exposed to particularly high concentrations of nitrogen dioxide. Therefore, individuals with heart or respiratory disease should avoid prolonged exposure to high-traffic areas and in-home heating devices that are unventilated.

Carbon Monoxide—A Deadly Gas

Carbon monoxide (CO), a colorless, odorless, and very toxic gas, occurs widely in the environment. It is found in fumes from cars and trucks. It is also produced by generators, stoves, lanterns, burning charcoal and wood, gas ranges, and heating systems.

During exposure to carbon monoxide, the gas enters your lungs and binds tightly to hemoglobin, the red, oxygen-carrying protein pigment in your red blood cells. Carbon monoxide literally pushes oxygen off your red blood cells. Carbon monoxide in any concentration is harmful to the body, especially to the heart and brain.

High concentrations of carbon monoxide can kill or seriously injure a person within minutes. For example, motor boaters have succumbed to the odorless gas while attending to a running engine underneath a wharf. Chronic, low-level exposure to carbon monoxide can cause serious respiratory disease and shorten your life. Smoking tobacco and breathing tobacco smoke raises carbon monoxide levels in your blood, eventually causing disease.

Even seemingly incidental exposure to carbon monoxide from generator, motorboat, ski-boat, or houseboat exhausts can produce

dangerous levels of carbon monoxide in the blood. In poorly venti-
lated parking structures, carbon monoxide can create problems for
people who have atherosclerotic disease or other cardiac conditions.

Centers for Disease Control and Prevention Guidelines for Carbon Monoxide

The CDC suggests preventing exposure to carbon monoxide with these precautions:

- Have your heating system, water heater, and any other gas-, oil-, or coal-burning appliances serviced by a qualified technician annually.

- Install a battery-operated carbon monoxide detector in your home and check or replace the battery regularly. In the event the detector is activated, leave your home immediately and call 911.

- Seek prompt medical attention if you suspect you have carbon monoxide poisoning because you are feeling dizzy, light-headed, or nauseous.

- Avoid using a generator, charcoal grill, camp stove, or other gasoline- or charcoal-burning device inside your home, basement, or garage.

- Avoid operating a car or truck inside a garage attached to your house, even if you leave the door open.

- Avoid burning anything in a stove or fireplace that isn't vented.

- Avoid heating your house by means of your gas oven.

Sulfur Dioxide: A Highly Toxic Gas

Sulfur dioxide (SO_2) is a colorless gas with a pungent odor and taste.
When sulfur dioxide contacts the moisture in your eyes, nose, or
respiratory tract, it forms the highly irritating sulfurous acid.

Sulfur dioxide is discharged by many industrial processes as well
as volcanoes. For example, the combustion of coal and petroleum
compounds that contain sulfur generates sulfur dioxide. Sulfur
dioxide, especially in the presence of a catalyst such as nitrogen

dioxide, forms sulfuric acid in the form of acid rain. Sulfur dioxide easily combines with oxygen to form sulfur trioxide (SO_3), which quickly mixes with water to form sulfuric acid.

The concentration of sulfur dioxide in the air in your neighborhood is likely to be low, particularly indoors. On the other hand, an indoor kerosene space heater can emit a significant amount of sulfur dioxide into your house.

Ozone

Ozone (O_3) is a highly reactive, colorless-to-bluish gas with an almost-pleasant, characteristically sweet odor. We associate the odor of ozone with electrical motors or clothes dried in the sun. Ozone is created by radiation from the sun striking molecules of oxygen (O_2) in the stratosphere (a layer in the atmosphere about seven miles above the earth). Ozone prevents high-energy ultraviolet (UV) radiation from penetrating the earth's atmosphere and destroying most life forms. This high-altitude ozone is not harmful to human health as it is miles away and we do not breathe it. However, ozone may also form close to the ground through reactions between smog and sunlight. Low-altitude ozone is harmful and may be mixed with the air you breathe.

Low-level ozone exposure cannot be avoided because ozone is created by many natural processes and human activities. The concentration of ozone in the air around you varies with the time of day, temperature, and wind speed and direction.

A 2007 study involving one million US subjects showed that higher ozone levels increased the risk of cardiovascular death due to high temperatures. One explanation is that exposure to ozone may alter the respiratory airway and the autonomic (involuntary) nervous system, leaving individuals more vulnerable to the effects of fluctuations in temperature.

Some authorities recommend that environmental warnings during hot weather include information on ozone levels. The impact of ozone on health is likely to increase if global warming worsens.

Secondhand Smoke

Secondhand smoke, also referred to as environmental tobacco smoke, accounts for the majority of indoor air pollution whenever someone is smoking nearby. Studies of secondhand smoke have shown that it adversely affects the heart and circulatory system, probably by speeding the development of atherosclerosis or reducing the flexibility of coronary arteries by increasing their thickness.

Types of Heart Disease Aggravated by Air Pollution

There is strong evidence that even low doses of air pollution can adversely affect heart function, particularly in patients with established heart disease.

As noted earlier, patients with heart disease who are exposed to air pollution are more likely to require hospitalization or die. Particularly vulnerable patients include those with coronary atherosclerosis, congestive heart failure, or frequent heart rhythm irregularities.

Air pollution can have a negative effect on the heart that occurs either slowly or suddenly. For example, air pollution appears to promote long-term development of coronary atherosclerosis, which can lead to a possible heart attack. On the other hand, air pollution may promote an abrupt, deadly heart event, such as a sudden irregular heartbeat or heart attack.

These effects on the heart are sometimes exacerbated by the development of excessive stickiness of the particles in the blood that promote clot formation, called platelets. The effects can also be related to inflammation in arteries supplying blood to the heart muscle or by causing other damage to the inner lining of coronary arteries.

Significant Risk from Air Pollution

The contribution of air pollution to the risk of illness or death from heart disease is not as great as that associated with known cardiovascular risk factors such as cigarette smoking, diabetes, hypertension, or obesity. Still, the risk from air pollution is significant, partly due to the fact that many people experience a lifetime of exposure to air pollution.

Studies suggest that, in addition to people with underlying heart disease, those who are elderly, have lung disease or diabetes, or are of lower socioeconomic status are at particularly increased risk from air pollution.

The Air Quality Index and the Environmental Protection Agency

The Air Quality Index (AQI) is a rating that the Environmental Protection Agency (EPA) and other agencies use to alert the public about local air quality and related health concerns. The AQI addresses health effects that can occur within a few hours or days after breathing polluted air. AQI values range from 0 to 500, with 0–50, 100–200, and 300–500 representing "good," "unhealthy," and "hazardous" air quality, respectively.

Recent Studies

Recent studies on air pollution have shown that exposure to toxins or particulate matter in air pollution varies both within a city and between different cities.

- If you live near a major road you are more likely to develop hardening of the arteries or die of a cardiovascular event, such as a heart attack or irregular heart rhythm.

- The life of an individual living in a densely polluted US city could be shortened by 1.8 to 3.1 years due to chronic air pollution. About 70% of this shortened life span is due to cardiovascular causes.

- Exposure to high levels of diesel exhaust may interfere with normal blood vessel function and clotting activity.

Summary

Air pollution increases the risk of cardiovascular illness and death, particularly in urban and industrial areas, although the ways air pollution causes harmful effects are just now beginning to be understood. If you have pre-existing heart failure or coronary artery disease, you may want to talk with your doctor about the risks related to air pollution in their environment.

By Daniel Hayes, MD, April 2010.

Chapter 44

Questioning
Chelation Therapy

Chelation is a chemical process in which a substance is used to bind molecules, such as metals or minerals, and hold them tightly so they can be removed from a system, such as the body. In medicine, chelation has been scientifically proven to rid the body of excess or toxic metals. For example, a person who has lead poisoning may be given chelation therapy in order to bind and remove excess lead from the body before it can cause damage.

Chelation therapy is usually performed with salts of EDTA, a synthetic, or man-made, amino acid delivered through the veins. EDTA was first used in the 1940s for the treatment of heavy metal poisoning. Calcium disodium EDTA chelation removes heavy metals and minerals, such as lead, iron, copper, and calcium, from the blood and is approved by the FDA for use in treating lead poisoning and toxicity from other heavy metals.

Both calcium disodium EDTA and disodium EDTA are commonly referred to as EDTA. Although similarly named, they appear to differ significantly in their safety profile. Calcium EDTA is approved for severe lead poisoning and appears to be the safer of the two drugs. Disodium EDTA is not approved for lead poisoning and appears to carry significantly greater risks.

Calcium is one of the substances that forms the plaque of atherosclerosis. It is possible to remove calcium from the body through EDTA chelation, which has led some to speculate that chelation therapy could be used to treat atherosclerosis. Some alternative medicine practitioners advocate and perform EDTA chelation therapy for atherosclerosis, despite little research on this use.

Several small studies have examined chelation therapy for atherosclerosis and found no evidence of success. However, proponents of chelation therapy have argued the studies were too small to detect a benefit. The agencies of the NIH have launched the Trial to Assess Chelation Therapy (TACT) to assess the effectiveness of this therapy in a larger number of patients. Most chelation therapy practitioners use disodium EDTA, rather than calcium disodium EDTA. For this reason, TACT uses disodium EDTA under an FDA license as an investigational new drug (IND).

EDTA Chelation Therapy Side Effects

In 2008, the FDA issued a public health advisory regarding disodium EDTA. The FDA has received multiple reports of deaths in patients administered disodium EDTA, in most cases given in error instead of calcium EDTA. The FDA is currently considering whether the benefits of disodium EDTA exceed its risks and if it should remain on the market.

The most common side effect is a burning sensation at the site where the EDTA was delivered into the vein. Rare side effects can include fever, headache, nausea, and vomiting. Even more rare are serious and potentially fatal side effects that can include heart failure, a sudden drop in blood pressure, abnormally low calcium levels in the blood, permanent kidney damage, and bone marrow depression (meaning blood cell counts fall). Reversible injury to the kidneys, although infrequent, has been reported with EDTA chelation therapy. Other serious side effects can occur if EDTA is not administered by a trained health professional. As noted earlier, there are a number of reports of deaths resulting from the use of disodium EDTA, including by alternative medicine practitioners.

Theories about EDTA Chelation Therapy and Blocked Arteries

Those who recommend chelation therapy have suggested several ideas. One idea suggests EDTA chelation might work by directly removing calcium found in fatty plaque blocking the arteries, causing the plaque deposits to break up. Another theory assumes the process of chelation may stimulate the release of a hormone that, in turn, causes calcium to be removed from plaque or causes a lowering of cholesterol levels. A third idea is that EDTA chelation therapy may work by reducing the damaging effects of oxygen ions (oxidative stress) on the walls of the blood vessels. Reducing oxidative stress could reduce inflammation in the arteries and improve blood vessel function. None of these ideas has been well tested in scientific studies.

Lack of Evidence that EDTA Chelation Therapy Works for Coronary Artery Disease

At this point, there is little scientific evidence that chelation therapy is effective for coronary artery disease (CAD). Virtually all published data supporting the benefits of chelation therapy are from individual case reports and series by chelation therapy practitioners. The validity of these reports has been questioned on several different points. Most did not use consistent methods, and few used any objective measures of improvement. The case reports also have not compared the effects of chelation against placebos (inert sham treatments where patients believe they are receiving chelation therapy but do not actually receive EDTA). These shortcomings make it difficult to determine whether reported effects were actually due to treatment.

A total of six published controlled studies have looked at chelation therapy for cardiovascular disease. A 1991 study by Dr. Sloth-Nielsen's research group found no difference in angiogram results in 30 patients who received either chelation therapy or a placebo. A 1994 study by Dr. Van Rij's research group found no differences on several measures of peripheral vascular disease among 32 patients who received either chelation treatments or a placebo. Two additional studies by Dr. Guldager's research group in 1992 found no differences after treatment between groups in cholesterol profiles, treadmill performance, or several other measures.

The only study to report improvement with chelation therapy was a 1990 study by Dr. Olszewer's research group. However, it has been considered a poor-quality study since it involved only 10 patients and did not have a control group. The authors reported improvement in treated patients but did not publish sufficient data for others to assess whether their conclusions were accurate.

The best evidence so far comes from a 2002 study known as PATCH (Program to Assess Alternative Treatment Strategies to Achieve Cardiac Health). This Canadian study examined 84 patients with confirmed CAD. Half received EDTA chelation therapy, and the other half received a matching placebo solution. Seventy-eight patients completed the trial and were assessed by EKG treadmill testing before and after 27 weeks of treatment. There were no differences in outcomes between the two groups at the end of the study. A second study looking at some of these same patients found no improvement in measures of blood vessel function between the two groups.

While controlled studies have been almost uniformly negative, chelation therapy advocates have argued these studies involved too few patients to rule out a benefit. In 2003, the NIH began a five-year study known as TACT to determine whether chelation therapy is effective for cardiovascular disease. The study was intended to enroll 2,000 participants, which it was hoped would provide definitive evidence.

However, in 2008, a scientific group lead by Dr. Kimball Atwood at the Tufts University School of Medicine published a blistering attack on the TACT study. They provided a detailed analysis of the study and its history and accused the trial's organizers of unethical and improper behavior. The article alleged that many TACT investigators had improper qualifications, histories of professional and scientific misconduct, or conflicts of interest that would bias outcomes. They also argued that patients were not given accurate information regarding potential risks of treatment. The authors believed any results from TACT would be unreliable and that the study should be abandoned.

Later in 2008, enrollment in the TACT study was halted largely due to the criticisms from Dr. Atwood's group. Safety reviewers expressed concern that the study's consent forms for patients contained misrepresentations. However, the TACT was allowed to proceed with the patients who had already been enrolled.

One week prior to TACT's enrollment suspension, a second NIH study of chelation therapy for autism was cancelled. At issue were the same concerns about information given to participants as well as new animal data suggesting chelation therapy could cause brain damage.

Results of the TACT study are expected in 2010, but due to these controversies it is far from clear whether this will be the final word on the subject.

Excerpted and adapted from "Questions and Answers: The NIH Trial of EDTA Chelation Therapy for Coronary Artery Disease," June 2004, and "Learn More about Chelation Therapy and the Study," October 2009, both produced by the National Center for Complementary and Alternative Medicine (NCCAM, nccam.nih.gov). Revised, updated, and expanded by David A. Cooke MD, FACP April 2010.

Chapter 45

Finding Recipes for Heart Health

Cookbooks with Heart-Healthy Recipes

The 300 Calorie Cookbook by the editors of Betty Crocker. Published by Betty Crocker, 2009. ISBN: 0470080590.

365 Days of Healthy Eating by the American Dietetic Association. Published by Wiley, 2003. ISBN: 0471442216.

500 Low-Sodium Recipes by Dick Logue. Published by Fair Winds Press, 2007. ISBN: 1592332773.

All Heart Family Cookbook by WomenHeart: The National Coalition for Women with Heart Disease. Published by Rodale Books, 2007. ISBN: 1594867968.

The Complete Idiot's Guide to Low-Salt Meals by Shelly James and Heidi McIndoo. Published by Alpha, 2006. ISBN: 159257467X.

The DASH Diet Action Plan by Marla Heller. Published by Amidon Press, 2007. ISBN: 097634081X.

The DASH Diet for Hypertension by Thomas Moore and Mark Jenkins. Published by Pocket, 2003. ISBN: 0743410076.

Diabetes and Heart Healthy Meals for Two by the American Diabetes Association and the American Heart Association. Published by the American Heart Association, 2008. ISBN: 1580403050.

Eat to Beat High Blood Pressure by the editors of Reader's Digest. Published by Reader's Digest, 2007. ISBN: 0762108983.

Eat, Drink, and Be Healthy: The Harvard Medical School Guide to Healthy Eating by Walter Willett. Published by Free Press, 2005. ISBN: 0743266420.

Eating for Lower Cholesterol by Catherine Jones and Elaine Trujillo. Published by Da Capo Press, 2005. ISBN: 156924376X.

The EatingWell for a Healthy Heart Cookbook by Philip Ades and the editors of *EatingWell Magazine*. Published by Countryman, 2008. ISBN: 0881507245.

Everyday Cooking with Dean Ornish by Dean Ornish. Published by Harper Perennial, 1996. ISBN: 0060928115.

The Everything Low-Cholesterol Cookbook by Linda Larsen. Published by Adams Media, 2008. ISBN: 1598694014.

Healthy Family Meals by the American Heart Association. Published by Clarkson Potter, 2009. ISBN: 0307450597.

Healthy Heart Cookbook by the editors of Betty Crocker. Published by Betty Crocker, 2004. ISBN: 0764574248.

The Healthy Heart Cookbook for Dummies by James Rippe. Published by For Dummies, 2000. ISBN: 0764552228.

The Healthy Heart Cookbook: Over 700 Recipes for Every Day and Every Occasion by Joseph Piscatella and Bernie Piscatella. Published by Black Dog & Leventhal Publishers, 2003. ISBN: 1579123309.

Heart Healthy Lifestyle Guide and Cookbook by the Cleveland Clinic Heart Center. Published by Broadway, 2007. ISBN: 0767921682.

Hypertension Cookbook by Karen Levin and the American Medical Association. Published by the American Medical Association, 2005. ISBN: 0696224437.

Keep the Beat Recipes by the National Heart, Lung, and Blood Institute. Published by the National Institutes of Health, 2009. ISBN: 1933236159.

Low-Calorie Cookbook by the American Heart Association. Published by Clarkson Potter, 2004. ISBN: 0812928555.

Low-Cholesterol Cookbook for Dummies by Molly Siple. Published by For Dummies, 2004. ISBN: 0764571605.

Low-Fat and Luscious Desserts by the American Heart Association. Published by Clarkson Potter, 2000. ISBN: 0812933362.

Low-Fat, Low-Cholesterol Cookbook, Fourth Edition, by the American Heart Association. Published by Clarkson Potter, 2010. ISBN: 030758755X.

Low-Fat, Low-Cholesterol Cooking by the editors of Betty Crocker. Published by Betty Crocker, 2000. ISBN: 0028637623.

Low-Salt Cookbook, Third Edition, by the American Heart Association. Published by Clarkson Potter, 2007. ISBN: 1400097622.

Meals in Minutes Cookbook by the American Heart Association. Published by Clarkson Potter, 2002. ISBN: 0609809776.

The New American Heart Association Cookbook, Seventh Edition, by the American Heart Association. Published by Clarkson Potter, 2007. ISBN: 0307352056.

The New Mediterranean Diet Cookbook by Nancy Harmon Jenkins. Published by Bantam, 2008. ISBN: 0553385097.

No-Fad Diet: A Personal Plan for Healthy Weight Loss by the American Heart Association. Published by Clarkson Potter, 2006. ISBN: 0307347427.

One-Dish Meals by the American Heart Association. Published by Clarkson Potter, 2004. ISBN: 140008184X.

Prevent and Reverse Heart Disease by Caldwell Esselstyn. Published by Avery Trade, 2008. ISBN: 1583333002.

Quick and Easy Cookbook by the American Heart Association. Published by Clarkson Potter, 2001. ISBN: 0609808621.

The What to Eat If You Have Heart Disease Cookbook by Daniella Chace. Published by Contemporary Books, 2000. ISBN: 0809297094.

Websites with Heart-Healthy Recipes

AllRecipes.com
allrecipes.com/Info/Healthy-Cooking/Heart-Healthy/Main.aspx

allrecipes.com/Recipes/Healthy-Cooking/Low-Fat/Main.aspx

American Heart Association
www.americanheart.org/presenter.jhtml?identifier=3056412

Centers for Disease Control and Prevention
apps.nccd.cdc.gov/dnparecipe/recipesearch.aspx

Diabetic Living
www.diabeticlivingonline.com/diabetic-recipes/low-cholesterol

FoodNetwork.com
www.foodnetwork.com/topics/low-cholesterol/index.html

www.foodnetwork.com/topics/low-sodium/index.html

Healing Heart Foundation
heart.kumu.org/recipes.html

Heart Healthy Living
www.hearthealthyonline.com

MayoClinic.com
www.mayoclinic.com/health/heart-healthy-recipes/re00098

www.mayoclinic.com/health/low-sodium-recipes/re00101

www.mayoclinic.com/health/low-fat-recipes/re00100

Mrs. Dash
www.mrsdash.com/recipes/recipe-search-results.aspx?list=Low-Sodium-Recipes

National Heart, Lung, and Blood Institute
www.nhlbi.nih.gov/health/public/heart/other/ktb_recipebk/ktb_recipebk.pdf

hp2010.nhlbihin.net/healthyeating/CategoryList.aspx

www.nhlbi.nih.gov/health/public/heart/hbp/dash/new_dash.pdf

Reader's Digest
www.rd.com/heart-healthy-recipes

West Virginia University
www.hsc.wvu.edu/Wellness/Wellness-Recipes/ornish_recipes/index_ornish_recipes.htm

Sample Recipes for Heart Health

Zucchini Lasagna
Say cheese because this healthy version of a favorite comfort food will leave you smiling.

Ingredients:

1/2 pound lasagna noodles, cooked in unsalted water	2 1/2 cups tomato sauce, no salt added
3/4 cup part-skim mozzarella cheese, grated	2 teaspoons basil, dried
	2 teaspoons oregano, dried
1 1/2 cups fat-free cottage cheese	1/4 cup onion, chopped
1/4 cup Parmesan cheese, grated	1 clove garlic
1 1/2 cups zucchini, raw, sliced	1/8 teaspoon black pepper

- Preheat oven to 350 degrees Fahrenheit. Lightly spray 9x13-inch baking dish with vegetable oil spray.

- In small bowl, combine 1/8 cup mozzarella and 1 tablespoon Parmesan cheese. Set aside.

- In medium bowl, combine remaining mozzarella and Parmesan cheese with all the cottage cheese. Mix well and set aside.

- Combine tomato sauce with remaining ingredients. Spread thin layer of tomato sauce in bottom of baking dish. Add one-third of the noodles in single layer. Spread half the cottage cheese mixture on top. Add layer of zucchini.

- Repeat layering.

- Add thin coating of sauce. Top with noodles, sauce, and reserved cheese mixture. Cover with aluminum foil.

- Bake for 30–40 minutes. Cool for 10–15 minutes. Cut into six portions.

Serving suggestion: Use unsalted cottage cheese to reduce the sodium content to 196 mg per serving.

Serving size: 1 piece; calories: 276; fat: 5 g; carbohydrates: 41 g; protein: 19 g; cholesterol: 11 mg; sodium: 380 mg.

Baked Salmon Dijon

This salmon entrée is easy to make and a delicious treat for family and friends.

Ingredients:

1 cup fat-free sour cream

2 teaspoons dried dill

3 tablespoons scallions, finely chopped

2 tablespoons Dijon mustard

2 tablespoons lemon juice

1 1/2 pounds salmon fillet with skin, cut in center

1/2 teaspoon garlic powder

1/2 teaspoon black pepper

Fat-free cooking spray, as needed

- Whisk sour cream, dill, onion, mustard, and lemon juice in small bowl to blend.

- Preheat oven to 400 degrees Fahrenheit. Lightly oil baking sheet with cooking spray.

- Place salmon, skin side down, on prepared sheet. Sprinkle with garlic powder and pepper. Spread with the sauce.

- Bake salmon until just opaque in center, about 20 minutes.

Serving size: 1 piece (4 ounces); calories: 196; fat: 7 g; carbohydrates: 5 g; protein: 27 g; cholesterol: 76 mg; sodium: 229 mg.

Barbecued Chicken

Fall under the spell of this Southern-style, sweet barbecue sauce.

Ingredients:

5 tablespoons (3 ounces) tomato paste

1 teaspoon ketchup

2 teaspoons honey

1 teaspoon molasses

1 teaspoon Worcestershire sauce

4 teaspoons white vinegar

3/4 teaspoon cayenne pepper

1/8 teaspoon black pepper

1/4 teaspoon onion powder

2 cloves garlic, minced

1/8 teaspoon ginger, grated

1 1/2 pounds chicken (breasts, drumsticks), skinless

- Combine all ingredients except chicken in saucepan. Simmer for 15 minutes.
- Wash chicken and pat dry. Place on large platter and brush with half the sauce mixture.
- Cover with plastic wrap and marinate in refrigerator for 1 hour.
- Place chicken on baking sheet lined with aluminum foil and broil for 10 minutes on each side to seal in juices.
- Turn down oven to 350 degrees Fahrenheit and add remaining sauce to chicken. Cover chicken with aluminum foil and continue baking for 30 minutes.

Serving size: 1/2 breast or 2 small drumsticks; calories: 176; fat: 4 g; carbohydrates: 7 g; protein: 27 g; cholesterol: 81 mg; sodium: 199 mg.

Stir-Fried Beef and Vegetables

Stir-frying uses very little oil, as this tasty dish shows.

Ingredients:

2 tablespoons dry red wine

1 tablespoon soy sauce

1/2 teaspoon sugar

1 1/2 teaspoons ginger root, peeled, grated

1 pound boneless round steak, fat trimmed and cut across grain into 1 1/2-inch strips

2 tablespoons vegetable oil

2 medium onions, each cut into 8 wedges

1/2 pound fresh mushrooms, rinsed, trimmed, and sliced

2 stalks celery, cut on the diagonal into 1/4-inch slices

2 small green peppers, cut into thin lengthwise strips

1 cup water chestnuts, drained, sliced

2 tablespoons cornstarch

1/4 cup water

- Prepare marinade by mixing wine, soy sauce, sugar, and ginger.
- Marinate meat in mixture while preparing vegetables.

- Heat 1 tablespoon oil in large skillet or wok. Stir-fry onions and mushrooms for 3 minutes over medium-high heat.

- Add celery and cook for 1 minute. Add remaining vegetables and cook for 2 minutes or until green pepper is tender but crisp. Transfer vegetables to warm bowl.

- Add remaining 1 tablespoon oil to skillet. Stir-fry meat in oil for about 2 minutes or until meat loses its pink color.

- Blend cornstarch and water. Stir into meat. Cook and stir until thickened.

- Return vegetables to skillet. Stir gently and serve.

Serving size: 6 ounces; calories: 179; fat: 7 g; carbohydrates: 12 g; protein: 17 g; cholesterol: 40 mg; sodium: 201 mg.

Classic Macaroni and Cheese

Here's a scrumptious, lower-fat version of a favorite dish.

Ingredients:

2 cups macaroni	1/4 teaspoon black pepper
1/2 cup onions, chopped	1 1/4 cups (4 ounces) low-fat sharp
1/2 cup evaporated skim milk	cheddar cheese, finely shredded
1 medium egg, beaten	Nonstick cooking spray, as needed

- Cook macaroni according to directions, but do not add salt to the cooking water. Drain and set aside.

- Spray casserole dish with nonstick cooking spray. Preheat oven to 350 degrees Fahrenheit.

- Lightly spray saucepan with nonstick cooking spray. Add onions and sauté for about 3 minutes.

- In another bowl, combine macaroni, onions, and rest of ingredients and mix.

- Transfer mixture into casserole dish.

- Bake for 25 minutes or until bubbly. Let stand for 10 minutes before serving.

Serving size: 1/2 cup; calories: 200; fat: 4 g; carbohydrates: 29 g; protein: 11 g; cholesterol: 34 mg; sodium: 120 mg.

Sweet Potato Custard

Sweet potatoes and bananas combine to make this flavorful, low-fat custard.

Ingredients:

1 cup sweet potato, cooked, mashed	2 egg yolks (or 1/3 cup egg substitute), beaten
1/2 cup banana (about 2 small), mashed	1/2 teaspoon salt
	1/4 cup raisins
1 cup evaporated skim milk	1 tablespoon sugar
2 tablespoons packed brown sugar	1 teaspoon ground cinnamon
	Nonstick cooking spray, as needed

- Preheat oven to 325 degrees Fahrenheit.
- In medium bowl, stir together sweet potato and banana. Add milk, blending well.
- Add brown sugar, egg yolks, and salt, mixing thoroughly.
- Spray 1-quart casserole with nonstick cooking spray. Transfer sweet potato mixture to casserole dish.
- Combine raisins, sugar, and cinnamon. Sprinkle over top of sweet potato mixture.
- Bake for 40–45 minutes or until knife inserted near center comes out clean.

Serving size: 1/2 cup; calories: 160; fat: 2 g; carbohydrates: 32 g; protein: 5 g; cholesterol: 72 mg; sodium: 255 mg. (Note: If using egg substitute, cholesterol will be lower.)

Apple Coffee Cake

Apples and raisins keep this cake delectably moist, using less oil and promoting heart health.

Ingredients:

5 cups tart apples, cored, peeled, chopped

1 cup sugar

1 cup dark raisins

1/2 cup pecans, chopped

1/4 cup vegetable oil

2 teaspoons vanilla

1 egg, beaten

2 cups all-purpose flour, sifted

1 teaspoon baking soda

2 teaspoons ground cinnamon

- Preheat oven to 350 degrees Fahrenheit. Lightly oil 13x9-inch pan.

- In large mixing bowl, combine apples with sugar, raisins, and pecans. Mix well and let stand for 30 minutes.

- Stir in oil, vanilla, and egg.

- Sift together flour, soda, and cinnamon and stir into apple mixture about a third at a time—just enough to moisten dry ingredients.

- Turn batter into pan. Bake for 35–40 minutes. Cool cake slightly before serving.

Serving size: 3 1/2-inch x 2 1/2-inch piece; calories: 196; fat: 8 g; carbohydrates: 31 g; protein: 3 g; cholesterol: 11 mg; sodium: 67 mg.

1–2–3 Peach Cobbler

Try this healthier, mouth-watering take on a classic favorite.

Ingredients:

1/2 teaspoon ground cinnamon

1 tablespoon vanilla extract

2 tablespoons cornstarch

1 cup peach nectar

1/4 cup pineapple or peach juice (can use juice from canned peaches)

2 cans (16 ounces each) peaches, packed in juice, drained, or 1 3/4 pound fresh, sliced

1 tablespoon tub margarine

1 cup dry pancake mix

2/3 cup all-purpose flour

1/2 cup sugar

2/3 cup evaporated skim milk

Nonstick cooking spray, as needed

1/2 teaspoon nutmeg

1 tablespoon brown sugar

- Combine cinnamon, vanilla, cornstarch, peach nectar, and pineapple or peach juice in saucepan over medium heat. Stir constantly until mixture thickens and bubbles.

- Add sliced peaches to mixture. Reduce heat and simmer for 5–10 minutes.

- In another saucepan, melt margarine and set aside.

- Lightly spray 8-inch square glass dish with cooking spray. Pour in peach mixture.

- In another bowl, combine pancake mix, flour, sugar, and melted margarine. Stir in milk. Quickly spoon this mixture over peach mixture.

- Combine nutmeg and brown sugar. Sprinkle mixture on top of batter.

- Bake at 400 degrees Fahrenheit for 15–20 minutes or until golden brown. Cool and cut into 8 squares.

Serving size: 1 square; calories: 271; fat: 4 g; carbohydrates: 54 g; protein: 4 g; cholesterol: less than 1 mg; sodium: 263 mg.

Recipes excerpted from "When Delicious Meets Nutritious: Recipes for Heart Health," National Heart, Lung, and Blood Institute (NHLBI, www.nhlbi.nih.gov), January 2005. Resources compiled by the editors, April 2010. Inclusion does not constitute endorsement, and there is no implication associated with omission.

Chapter 46

Directory of Heart Disease Organizations

Agency for Healthcare Research and Quality (AHRQ)

Office of Communications and Knowledge Transfer
540 Gaither Road, Suite 2000
Rockville, MD 20850
Phone: 301-427-1364
Fax: 301-427-1873
Website: www.ahrq.gov

The Agency for Healthcare Research and Quality (AHRQ) is committed to helping improve our health care system. AHRQ conducts and supports a wide range of health services research for clinicians, policymakers, purchasers, health plans, and health systems. AHRQ research helps consumers play an active role in their health care and reduces the likelihood they will be subject to a medical error by providing health care guides. Topics for consumers include "Staying Healthy," "Choosing Quality Care," "Getting Safer Care," "Understanding Diseases and Conditions," and "Comparing Medical Treatments."

American Academy of Family Physicians (AAFP)

P.O. Box 11210
Shawnee Mission, KS 66207-1210
Toll-Free: 800-274-2237
Phone: 913-906-6000
Fax: 913-906-6075
Website: www.aafp.org

The American Academy of Family Physicians (AAFP) is the national association of family doctors whose goal is to promote and maintain high-quality standards and comprehensive health care to the public. AAFP members enjoy free access to the full text of their journals and news publications. Content from *American Family Physician (AFP)* and *Family Practice Management (FPM)* that is more than 13 months old is available free of charge to the general public. Resources for cardiac patients can be found by searching for "Heart Disease" on the AAFP website.

American Academy of Pediatrics (AAP)

141 Northwest Point Boulevard
Elk Grove Village, IL 60007-1098
Phone: 847-434-4000
Fax: 847-434-8000
Website: www.aap.org
Website: www.healthychildren.org (for parents)
E-mail: kidsdocs@aap.org

The American Academy of Pediatrics (AAP) website contains general information for parents of children from birth through age 21. AAP is an organization of pediatricians committed to the attainment of optimal physical, mental, and social health and well-being for all infants, children, adolescents, and young adults. They offer general information related to child health and more specific information concerning pediatric issues. AAP offers information on their many programs and activities, policies and guidelines, publications, and other child health resources. If you're a parent, visit HealthyChildren.org, which offers updated health care information, guidance for parents and caregivers, interactive tools, and personalized content. Specific questions can be answered by clicking "Ask a Pediatrician."

American Academy of Physical Medicine and Rehabilitation (AAPM&R)

9700 West Bryn Mawr Avenue
Suite 200
Rosemont, IL 60018-5701
Phone: 847-737-6000
Fax: 847-737-6001
Website: www.aapmr.org
E-mail: info@aapmr.org

The American Academy of Physical Medicine and Rehabilitation (AAPM&R) is the national medical specialty society for physiatrists (physicians who specialize in physical medicine and rehabilitation.) AAPM&R serves its members and their patients and other health professionals by fostering excellence in physiatric practice, education, and research. AAPM&R publishes a scientific journal titled *PM&R* to keep its members abreast of the latest findings. AAPM&R also offers patients a listing of local Physical Medicine and Rehabilitation (PM&R) physicians.

American Association for Clinical Chemistry (AACC)

1850 K Street NW, Suite 625
Washington, DC 20006
Toll-Free: 800-892-1400
Fax: 202-887-5093
Website: www.aacc.org
E-mail: custserv@aacc.org

The American Association for Clinical Chemistry (AACC) is an international scientific and medical society of clinical laboratory professionals, physicians, research scientists, and other individuals involved with clinical chemistry and related disciplines. AACC provides leadership in advancing the practice and profession of clinical laboratory science and its application to health care. AACC's publication, *Clinical Chemistry*, is the most cited in the field, and they offer many programs addressing the scientific, clinical, technical, and management challenges facing laboratory professionals. AACC spearheaded the development of Lab Tests Online (www .labtestsonline.org), a unique consumer-education program.

American Association of Cardiovascular and Pulmonary Rehabilitation (AACVPR)

401 North Michigan Avenue
Suite 2200
Chicago, IL 60611
Phone: 312-321-5146
Fax: 312-673-6924
Website: www.aacvpr.org
E-mail: aacvpr@aacvpr.org

The American Association of Cardiovascular and Pulmonary Rehabilitation (AACVPR) is a multidisciplinary professional association dedicated to reducing morbidity, mortality, and disability from cardiovascular and pulmonary disease through education, prevention, rehabilitation, research, and disease management. AACVPR affiliates provide local programs with networking opportunities across the United States and publish the *Journal of Cardiopulmonary Rehabilitation and Prevention (JCRP)*, *Guidelines for Cardiac Rehabilitation Programs*, *Guidelines for Pulmonary Rehabilitation Programs*, *Cardiac Rehabilitation Resource Manual*, *News & Views*, as well as other publications. AACVPR offers patient resources on their website under the heading "Resources for Patients."

American College of Cardiology (ACC)

Heart House
2400 N Street NW
Washington, DC 20037
Toll-Free: 800-253-4636
Phone: 202-375-6000
Fax: 202-375-7000
Website: www.acc.org

The American College of Cardiology (AAC) provides their members with tools to improve their cardiovascular care and practice through easy-to-use products, programs, and services. ACC publishes *Journals of the American College of Cardiology (JACC), JACC Cardiovascular Interventions, JACC Cardiovascular Imaging*, and *Cardiology.* AAC also offers Cardiosource.com, an online resource for clinical cardiovascular information and news.

American College of Chest Physicians (ACCP)

3300 Dundee Road
Northbrook, IL 60062-2348
Toll-Free: 800-343-2227
Phone: 847-498-1400
Fax: 847-498-5460
Website: www.chestnet.org
Email: accp@chestnet.org

The American College of Chest Physicians (ACCP) is a leading resource for the improvement of cardiopulmonary health and critical care worldwide. ACCP promotes the prevention and treatment of diseases of the chest through leadership, education, research, and communication. ACCP publishes *CHEST*, which offers pertinent information relating to chest diseases. *CHEST* is considered the leading cardiopulmonary journal and is an essential resource for medical professionals wanting to stay updated in cardiopulmonary and critical care medicine.

American College of Emergency Physicians (ACEP)

P.O. Box 619911
Dallas, TX 75261-9911
Toll-Free: 800-798-1822
Phone: 972-550-0911
Fax: 972-580-2816
Website: www.acep.org
E-mail: membership@acep.org

The American College of Emergency Physicians (ACEP) is the leading continuing education source for emergency physicians and the primary information resource on developments in the specialty. ACEP offers an extensive selection of books, manuals, and serials for emergency medicine professionals. ACEP's clinical journal, *Annals of Emergency Medicine*, offers information on original research, clinical reports, case studies, practical methods and techniques, and opinions about emergency medicine. *ACEP News* provides up-to-date information on the practice environment, health system reform issues, college activities, and other topics of interest to its members.

American College of Sports Medicine (ACSM)

P.O. Box 1440
Indianapolis, IN 46206-1440
Phone: 317-637-9200
Fax: 317-634-7817
Website: www.acsm.org

The American College of Sports Medicine (ACSM) is an organization whose members work in a wide range of medical specialties, allied health professions, and scientific disciplines. ACSM offers information on the diagnosis, treatment, and prevention of sports-related injuries, and they promote and integrate scientific research, education, and practical applications of sports medicine and exercise science to maintain and enhance physical performance, fitness, health, and quality of life.

American Council on Exercise (ACE)

4851 Paramount Drive
San Diego, CA 92123
Toll-Free: 888-825-3636
Phone: 858-279-8227
Fax: 858-576-6564
Website: www.acefitness.org
E-mail: support@acefitness.org

The American Council on Exercise (ACE) is a nonprofit organization committed to enriching quality of life through safe and effective exercise and physical activity. ACE protects all segments of society against ineffective fitness products, programs, and trends through its ongoing public education, outreach and research. ACE sets certification and continuing education standards for fitness professionals and has become an established resource for both fitness professionals and consumers. ACE provides free comprehensive, unbiased, scientific research impacting the fitness industry to consumers and professionals.

American Diabetes Association (ADA)

1701 North Beauregard Street
Alexandria, VA 22311
Toll-Free: 800-342-2383
Website: www.diabetes.org
E-mail: AskADA@diabetes.org

The American Diabetes Association (ADA) strives to prevent diabetes, cure it, and improve the lives of everyone affected by the disease. ADA publishes many books and resources for people with diabetes and the health care professionals who treat them, including a monthly magazine called *Diabetes Forecast* for people with diabetes. They also offer these professional journals: *Diabetes*, *Diabetes Care*, and *Diabetes Spectrum*.

American Dietetic Association (ADA)

120 South Riverside Plaza
Suite 2000
Chicago, IL 60606-6995
Toll-Free: 800-877-1600
Phone: 312-899-0040
Website: www.eatright.org

The American Dietetic Association (ADA) serves as an advocate to its members by promoting optimal nutrition and well-being for all people. To find a list of nutrition professionals in your area, click on "Find a Nutrition Professional." ADA publishes a monthly newsletter, *ADA Courier*, and a professional journal, *The Journal of the American Dietetic Association*. ADA also publishes several books and provides other resources for consumers and professionals.

American Heart Association (AHA)

National Center
7272 Greenville Avenue
Dallas, TX 75231
Toll-Free: 800-AHA-USA-1 (800-242-8721)
Website: www.americanheart.org
Website: www.hearthub.org (for patients)
E-mail: Review.personal.info@heart.org

The American Heart Association (AHA) is a nonprofit organization, and its goal is to reduce disability and death from heart disease and stroke through education. AHA offers HeartHub for patients, an online portal of information, tools, and resources about cardiovascular disease and stroke. Visit the Health Centers area of the HeartHub website to find a variety of articles and resources and videos. Professionals can connect with one another through AHA's Professional Online Network.

American Medical Women's Association (AMWA)

100 North 20th Street
Fourth Floor
Philadelphia, PA 19103
Phone: 215-320-3716
Fax: 215-564-2175
Website: www.amwa-doc.org

The American Medical Women's Association (AMWA) is an organization that functions at the local, national, and international levels to advance women in medicine and improve women's health. To accomplish this goal, AMWA provides and develops leadership through advocacy, education, expertise, mentoring, and strategic alliances. AMWA keeps members informed on issues that affect their practices and the health of their patients through a variety of electronic and print publications. AMWA's biweekly *Newsflash* updates members on advocacy issues and offers up-to-date health and professional information; *Connections*, a quarterly e-newsletter, features timely commentary on the issues that matter most to women physicians; and AMWA's official journal, *Journal of Women's Health*, provides a multidisciplinary approach and complete coverage of the latest advancements in the full purview of women's health care issues.

American Society of Echocardiography (ASE)

2100 Gateway Centre Boulevard
Suite 310
Morrisville, NC 27560
Phone: 919-861-5574
Fax: 919-882-9900
Website: www.asecho.org

The American Society of Echocardiography (ASE) is an organization of professionals committed to excellence in cardiovascular ultrasound and its application to patient care through education, advocacy, research, innovation, and service to its members and the public. ASE uses ultrasound to offer an exceptional view of the cardiovascular system to enhance patient care. Their goal is to raise public awareness of cardiovascular ultrasound through outreach campaigns that highlight the important role ultrasound plays in disease evaluation and management.

American Society of Hypertension, Inc. (ASH)

148 Madison Avenue, Fifth Floor
New York, NY 10016
Phone: 212-696-9099
Fax: 212-696-0711
Website: www.ash-us.org
E-mail: ash@ash-us.org

The American Society of Hypertension, Inc. (ASH) is the largest United States professional organization of scientific investigators and health care professionals committed to eliminating hypertension and its consequences for patients. ASH serves as a scientific forum bridging research with effective clinical treatment strategies. To find out more about hypertension, click on "About Hypertension" on the ASH website home page.

American Society of Nuclear Cardiology (ASNC)

4550 Montgomery Avenue, Suite 780 North
Bethesda, MD 20814-3304
Phone: 301-215-7575
Fax: 301-215-7113
Website: www.asnc.org
E-mail: info@asnc.org

The American Society of Nuclear Cardiology (ASNC) is a professional, not-for-profit organization that provides its members with a variety of continuing medical education programs related to nuclear cardiology and cardiovascular computed tomography (CT). ASNC is comprised of physicians, scientists, technologists, computer specialists, and other personnel working in the nuclear cardiology field. ASNC is international in scope with several hundred members residing in countries other than the United States.

American Stroke Association

National Center
7272 Greenville Avenue
Dallas, TX 75231
Toll-Free: 888-478-7653
Website: www.strokeassociation.org

The American Stroke Association provides effective, credible information for professional, patient, and general public audiences, with a specific emphasis on those at risk for stroke through research, education, fund raising, and advocacy. The American Stroke Association has many educational resources available online for consumers, including "Warning Signs," "Learn about Stroke," "Life after Stroke," and a "Heart and Stroke Encyclopedia." The American Stroke Association also offers "Seven Simple Steps to Live Better," which provides a personal heart score and a custom plan for living a healthy life.

Centers for Disease Control and Prevention (CDC)

1600 Clifton Road
Atlanta, GA 30333
Toll-Free: 800-CDC-INFO (800-232-4636)
Phone: 404-639-3311
TTY: 888-232-6348
Website: www.cdc.gov
E-mail: cdcinfo@cdc.gov

The Centers for Disease Control and Prevention (CDC) is dedicated to protecting health and promoting quality of life through the prevention and control of disease, injury, and disability. CDC offers a resource called "Division for Heart Disease and Stroke Prevention" that provides a list of CDC websites dealing with cardiovascular disease. Other resources for patients and professionals include "Learning about Heart Diseases," "Facts and Statistics," and "Education Materials."

Centers for Medicare and Medicaid Services (CMS)

7500 Security Boulevard
Baltimore, MD 21244-1850
Toll-Free: 800-633-4227
TTY/TTD: 877-486-2048
Website: www.medicare.gov

The Centers for Medicare and Medicaid Services (CMS) is a branch of the U.S. Department of Health and Human Services. CMS is the federal agency that administers the Medicare program and monitors the Medicaid programs offered by each state. English- and Spanish-speaking customer service representatives (CSRs) can answer questions and give information about Medicare coverage and costs, health plan options, and Medicare claims. CSRs are also available to order Medicare publications; help compare Medicare health plans, Medigap policies, and prescription drug plans; answer questions about claims and other insurance coverage; check eligibility for certain preventive services; give referrals; help find participating Medicare providers; and help find and compare hospitals, home health agencies, nursing homes, and dialysis facilities.

Children's Cardiomyopathy Foundation (CCF)

P.O. Box 547
Tenafly, NJ 07670
Phone: 866-808-2873

Fax: 201-227-7016
Website: www.childrenscardiomyopathy.org
E-mail: info@childrenscardiomyopathy.org

The Children's Cardiomyopathy Foundation (CCF) is a not-for-profit public charity and is the only organization in the country whose primary focus is pediatric cardiomyopathy. CCF plans to be a funding partner and the primary advocate for studies into the causes, diagnosis, treatment, and cure of pediatric cardiomyopathy. CCF actively works with federal agencies, medical societies, voluntary health organizations, and hospitals nationwide. Resources include news, facts about the disease, research, and support services.

Congenital Heart Information Network

101 North Washington Avenue, Suite 1A
Margate City, NJ 08402-1195
Phone: 609-822-1572
Fax: 609-822-1574
Website: www.tchin.org

The Congenital Heart Information Network is a national organization that provides reliable information, support services, financial assistance, and resources to families of children with congenital heart defects and acquired heart disease, adults with congenital heart defects, and the professionals who work with them. Resources include book reviews, support groups, and an extensive "Resource Room."

Heart Failure Society of America, Inc. (HFSA)

Court International, Suite 240 S
2550 University Avenue West
Saint Paul, MN 55114
Phone: 651-642-1633
Fax: 651-642-1502

Website: www.hfsa.org
E-mail: info@hfsa.org

The Heart Failure Society of America, Inc. (HFSA) is the first organized effort by heart failure experts from the Americas to provide a forum for those interested in heart function, heart failure, and congestive heart failure (CHF) research and patient care. HFSA strives to promote research related to all aspects of heart failure; to provide a forum for presentation of basic, clinical, and population-based research; to educate health care professionals through programs and publications to help them diagnose and treat heart failure; to serve as a resource for government, private industry, and health care providers; to enhance the quality and duration of life in those with heart failure; and to promote and facilitate the formal training of physicians, scientists, and health care providers in the field of heart failure.

Heart Rhythm Society

1400 K Street NW
Suite 500
Washington, DC 20005
Phone: 202-464-3400
Fax: 202-464-3401
Website: www.hrsonline.org
E-mail: info@hrsonline.org

The Heart Rhythm Society focuses on the science of and education and advocacy for cardiac arrhythmia professionals and patients. It has become the primary information resource on heart rhythm disorders, and its mission is to improve the care of patients by promoting research, education, and optimal health care policies and standards. *HeartRhythm*, the official journal of the Heart Rhythm Society, can be accessed online and includes podcast interviews. The "Patient Information" section of their website offers information about cardiac arrhythmia disorders.

Howard Gilman Institute for Heart Valve Disease

635 Madison Avenue, Third Floor
New York, NY 10022
Phone: 212-289-7777
Website: www.gilmanheartvalve.us
E-mail: info@gilmanheartvalve.us

The Howard Gilman Institute for Heart Valve Disease helps cardiologists, cardiothoracic surgeons, and other physicians take advantage of the most current concepts in evaluation and treatment of heart valve diseases. The Institute works hand-in-hand with medical professionals to take advantage of cutting-edge research and technology and provide the highest level of patient care. Patient care includes evaluation; synthesizing data from patient's history, physical examination, and test results; finding a diagnosis; recommending a course of treatment; implementing the treatment; and using the data to create new knowledge to achieve better future diagnosis and treatment.

Hypertrophic Cardiomyopathy Association (HCMA)

328 Green Pond Road
P.O. Box 306
Hibernia, NJ 07842
Phone: 973-983-7429
Fax: 973-983-7870
Website: www.4hcm.org
E-mail: support@4hcm.org

The Hypertrophic Cardiomyopathy Association (HCMA) is a not-for-profit organization that provides information, support, and advocacy to patients, their families, and medical providers in the area of hypertrophic cardiomyopathy (HCM). HCMA has several resources available to patients and their families, including an overview of the condition, "Symptoms," "Screening and Diagnosis," "Genetics," "Treatment," "Complications," "Research," and more.

March of Dimes

1275 Mamaroneck Avenue
White Plains, NY 10605
Phone: 914-997-4488
Website: www.marchofdimes.com

March of Dimes researchers, volunteers, educators, outreach workers, and advocates strive to improve the health of babies by preventing birth defects, premature birth, and infant mortality through research, community services, education, and advocacy. Articles on heart disease and heart defects can be found by searching for "Heart Disease" on the March of Dimes website.

Mended Hearts, Inc.

7272 Greenville Avenue
Dallas, TX 75231-4596
Toll-Free: 888-432-7899
Phone: 214-360-6149
Fax: 214-360-6145
Website: www.mendedhearts.org
E-mail: info@mendedhearts.org

Mended Hearts is a national nonprofit organization affiliated with the American Heart Association. It is recognized for its role in facilitating a positive patient-care experience. Mended Hearts partners offer services to heart patients through visiting programs, support group meetings, and educational forums. Educational online resources include "Dealing with Heart Disease," "Learn More about Heart Disease," archived articles from *Heartbeat* magazine, and links to other related resources.

Minneapolis Heart Institute Foundation (MHIF)

920 East 28th Street, Suite 100
Minneapolis, MN 55407

Toll-Free: 877-800-2729
Phone: 612-863-3833
Fax: 612-863-3801
Website: www.mplsheart.org
E-mail: info@mhif.org

The Minneapolis Heart Institute Foundation (MHIF) strives to promote and improve cardiovascular health, quality of life, and longevity. MHIF treats more cardiovascular patients using adult stem cell therapy than any other center in the nation, diagnoses cardiovascular disease at progressively earlier stages using noninvasive imaging, explores minimally invasive treatment options for patients with valve disease, investigates instances of sudden death on the athletic field and provides youth with tools to take an active role in their health, trains health professionals on the latest research, educates women wanting to lower their risk of heart disease, and improves access to health education and support networks through web-based programs and online communities. MHIF offers a list of "Community Programs and Services" on their website.

National Center for Complementary and Alternative Medicine (NCCAM)

National Institutes of Health
NCCAM Clearinghouse
P.O. Box 7923
Gaithersburg, MD 20898
Toll-Free: 888-644-6226
TTY: 866-464-3615
Fax: 866-464-3616
Website: nccam.nih.gov
E-mail: info@nccam.nih.gov

The National Center for Complementary and Alternative Medicine (NCCAM) is the government's lead agency for scientific research on the diverse medical and health care systems, practices, and products that are not generally considered part of conventional medicine. NCCAM offers several resources on heart health and heart disease by searching for "Heart Health" on their website. Information on clinical trials and research is also available on the website.

National Heart, Lung, and Blood Institute (NHLBI)

P.O. Box 30105
Bethesda, MD 20824-0105
Phone: 301-592-8573
TTY: 240-629-3255
Fax: 240-629-3246
Website: www.nhlbi.nih.gov
E-mail: nhlbiinfo@nhlbi.nih.gov

The National Heart, Lung, and Blood Institute (NHLBI) provides leadership in research, training, and education to promote the prevention and treatment of heart, lung, and blood diseases. NHLBI creates and supports a large, collaborative research base with private and public organizations, including academic institutions, industry, and other government agencies. NHLBI collaborates with patients, families, health care professionals, scientists, professional societies, patient advocacy groups, community organizations, and the media to promote the application of research results and leverage resources to address public health needs. Cardiovascular health information can be accessed on the site by searching for "Heart Health" or "Heart Disease." The website also offers information on clinical trials, news, and events of interest.

National Human Genome Research Institute

Communications and Public Liaison Branch
National Institutes of Health
Building 31
Room 4B09
31 Center Drive, MSC 2152
9000 Rockville Pike

Bethesda, MD 20892-2152
Phone: 301-402-0911
Fax: 301-402-2218
Website: www.genome.gov

The National Human Genome Research Institute was established to map the human genome. Today, genome technologies are used to study specific diseases, such as heart disease. Search for "Heart" for an extensive list of articles, presentations, and reports to get information on genome technology as it relates to heart disease and heart health.

National Hypertension Association (NHA)

324 East 30th Street
New York, NY 10016
Phone: 212-889-3557
Fax: 212-447-7032
Website: www.nathypertension.org
E-mail: nathypertension@aol.com

National Hypertension Association (NHA) research has focused mainly on a tumor called pheochromocytoma, which causes hypertension, and also on the mechanism of salt-induced hypertension. NHA has published extensively on these two topics, and two of its publications include *Our Greatest Threats: Live Longer, Live Better* and *100 Questions and Answers about Hypertension*. NHA also created a program, Values Initiative Teaching about Lifestyle (VITAL), in an effort to combat childhood obesity and high blood pressure. This program teaches healthy nutrition choices and appropriate physical activities to young school children (ages four through eight).

National Institute of Diabetes and Digestive and Kidney Diseases (NIDDK)

National Institute of Health
Building 31

Room 9A06
31 Center Drive, MSC 2560
Bethesda, MD 20892-2560
Phone: 301-496-3583
Website: www.niddk.nih.gov

The National Institute of Diabetes and Digestive and Kidney Diseases (NIDDK) conducts and supports research on serious diseases affecting public health. NIDDK supports much of the clinical research on the diseases of internal medicine and related subspecialty fields as well as many basic science disciplines. Its research encompasses the broad spectrum of metabolic diseases such as diabetes, obesity, inborn errors of metabolism, endocrine disorders, mineral metabolism, digestive and liver diseases, nutrition, urology and renal disease, and hematology. Various resources are available to consumers by searching for "Heart Health."

National Institute of Neurological Disorders and Stroke (NINDS)

NIH Neurological Institute
P.O. Box 5801
Bethesda, MD 20824
Toll-Free: 800-352-9424
Phone: 301-496-5751
TTY: 301-468-5981
Website: www.ninds.nih.gov

The National Institute of Neurological Disorders and Stroke (NINDS) strives to reduce the burden of neurological disease by conducting, coordinating, and guiding research on the causes, prevention, diagnosis, and treatment of neurological disorders and stroke and supports basic research in related scientific areas. NINDS also provides grants related to its areas of interest and collects and disseminates research information related to neurological disorders.

National Library of Medicine (NLM)

8600 Rockville Pike
Bethesda, MD 20894
Toll-Free: 888-346-3656
Phone: 301-594-5983
TDD: 800-735-2258
Fax: 301-402-1384
Website: www.nlm.nih.gov
E-mail: custserv@nlm.nih.gov

The National Library of Medicine (NLM) is the world's largest medical library. NLM collects materials and provides information and research services in all areas of biomedicine and health care. Online resources include MedlinePlus, *MedlinePlus Magazine*, current health news, online exhibitions, and a searchable database on heart disease and heart health topics.

National Stroke Association

9707 East Easter Lane
Centennial, CO 80112
Toll-Free: 800-STROKES (800-787-6537)
Fax: 303-649-1328
Website: www.stroke.org
E-mail: info@stroke.org

The National Stroke Association focuses 100% of its efforts on stroke, striving to lower the incidence and impact of stroke by developing compelling community outreach programs, calling for continued improvement in the quality of stroke patient care, and educating both health care professionals and the general public about stroke. Resources offered by the National Stroke Association include information on strokes, the risk factors associated with strokes, preventing strokes, and recovering from a stroke. Topics covered include "Stroke Survivors," "Caregivers and Families," "Women and Stroke," "African Americans and Stroke," and "Kids and Stroke."

Society for Vascular Surgery (SVS)

633 North St. Clair, 24th Floor
Chicago, IL 60611
Toll-Free: 800-258-7188
Phone: 312-334-2300
Fax: 312-334-2320
Website: www.vascularsociety.org
E-mail: vascular@vascularsociety.org

The Society for Vascular Surgery (SVS) seeks to advance excellence and innovation in vascular health through education, advocacy, research, and public awareness. SVS offers resources for medical professionals, patients, and their families. Consumer resources include "Information on Vascular Conditions, Tests, and Treatments" and "Find a Specialist."

Society of Thoracic Surgeons (STS)

633 North Saint Clair Street, Suite 2320
Chicago, IL 60611
Phone: 312-202-5800
Fax: 312-202-5801
Website: www.sts.org
E-mail: sts@sts.org

The Society of Thoracic Surgeons (STS) is a not-for-profit organization representing surgeons, researchers, and health professionals worldwide. It is STS's goal to enhance the ability of cardiothoracic surgeons to provide the highest quality patient care through education, research, and advocacy. Use the "Locate a Surgeon" resource to find surgeons by country or state.

Sudden Arrhythmia Death Syndromes Foundation (SADS)

508 East South Temple, Suite #20
Salt Lake City, UT 84102

Toll-Free: 800-STOP-SAD (800-786-7723)

Website: www.sads.org

The Sudden Arrhythmia Death Syndromes Foundation (SADS) is dedicated to informing the general public and medical professionals about the effects of untreated and undiagnosed cardiac arrhythmias and the methods by which death can be prevented. Initiatives include sponsoring public awareness meetings in local communities, providing educational videos, and establishing media relationships to promote publicity. SADS offers patient and family support resources and other educational resources including genetic testing information on their website.

Sudden Cardiac Arrest Association (SCAA)

1133 Connecticut Avenue NW, 11th Floor

Washington, DC 20036

Toll-Free: 866-972-7222

Fax: 202-719-8959

Website: www.suddencardiacarrest.org

E-mail: info@suddencardiacarrest.org

The Sudden Cardiac Arrest Association (SCAA) is an organization focused on sudden cardiac arrest. SCAA unites survivors, those at risk of sudden cardiac arrest, and others who are interested in being advocates. SCAA is dedicated to promoting solutions to help prevent sudden cardiac death, including increased awareness, immediate bystander action, public access to defibrillation (PAD), cardiovascular disease prevention, and access to preventative therapies. SCAA resources include videos, audio recordings, and interactive media as well as other educational materials including fact sheets, information on lab tests, and many other topics.

Texas Heart Institute

6770 Bertner Avenue

Houston, TX 77030

Phone: 832-355-4011

Website: www.texasheart.org

The Texas Heart Institute hopes to reduce the devastating toll of cardiovascular disease by providing a wealth of reliable information. Resources include patient care information, educational material on heart health, and heart disease risk factors.

U.S. Department of Health and Human Services (HHS)

200 Independence Avenue SW
Washington, DC 20201
Toll-Free: 877-696-6775
Website: www.hhs.gov

The Department of Health and Human Services (HHS) is the United States government's principal agency for protecting the health of all Americans and providing essential human services, especially for those who are least able to help themselves. Find information on health and disease, financial assistance, health insurance, safety, and statistics on the website.

U.S. Food and Drug Administration

10903 New Hampshire Avenue
Silver Spring, MD 20993
Toll-Free: 888-463-6332
Website: www.fda.gov

The Food and Drug Administration (FDA) is an agency within the U.S. Department of Health and Human Services. FDA is responsible for protecting public health by assuring the safety, effectiveness, and security of drugs, vaccines, biological products, medical devices, our nation's food supply, cosmetics, dietary supplements, and products that give off radiation. FDA also regulates tobacco products, advances public health by helping speed product innovations, and helps get the public accurate, science-based information to improve their health. Consumer FDA resources include information on eating for a healthy heart, heart health for women, heart disease, and many other topics. Search for "Heart Health" or "Heart Disease" for more information.

Vascular Disease Foundation (VDF)

1075 South Yukon
Suite 320
Lakewood, CO 80226
Toll-Free: 888-833-4463
Phone: 303-989-0500
Fax: 303-989-0200
Website: www.vdf.org

The Vascular Disease Foundation (VDF) strives to reduce death and disability from vascular diseases and improve vascular health. VDF increases public awareness and concern for vascular diseases and their impact on individuals, families, and society; provides information and educational programs for health care professionals; offers resources for public information related to vascular diseases; provides information and services to patients and their families; and helps patients and families affected by vascular diseases by creating patient advocacy and community support networks. Resources available on their website include disease information, news, events, fact sheets, "Find a Vascular Specialist," and more.

WomenHeart: The National Coalition for Women with Heart Disease

818 18th Street NW
Suite 1000
Washington, DC 20006
Toll-Free: 877-771-0030
Phone: 202-728-7199
Fax: 888-343-0764
Website: www.womenheart.org
E-mail: mail@womenheart.org

WomenHeart was founded by three women who had heart attacks while in their 40s. In addition to facing misdiagnosis and social isolation, they were surprised at how little information or services for women with heart disease were available. WomenHeart provides education, support, and hope by ensuring every woman has access to prevention, early detection, accurate diagnosis, and proper treatment. Website resources include "Support Services," "Heart Smart 101," "Living with Heart Disease," and "Prevention and Early Detection," among other topics.

Women's Heart Foundation (WHF)

P.O. Box 7827
West Trenton, NJ 08628
Phone: 609-771-9600
Fax: 609-771-3778
Website: www.womensheart.org

Women's Heart Foundation is a non-governmental organization that implements heart disease prevention projects. It is a coalition of executive nurses, civic leaders, community health directors, hospitals, women's heart centers, partners, providers, and corporate sponsors responding to women's heart disease. WHF advocates for women and supports early intervention and excellence in the care of women. Website information topics include "Exercise and Nutrition," "Heart Disease," and "Heart Surgery," as well as an "Ask the Nurse" option, a "PDF Library," and a glossary.

Compiled by the editors; inclusion does not constitute endorsement, and there is no implication associated with omission. All contact information verified in April 2010.

Index

Index

David A. Cooke, MD, FACP

David Cooke graduated Summa Cum Laude from Brandeis University in Massachusetts, and was elected to the Phi Beta Kappa honor society. Subsequently, he received his MD degree from the University of Michigan, where he was elected to the Alpha Omega Alpha medical honor society. After completing an internal medicine residency at the University of Wisconsin-Madison, he returned to Michigan. He is currently an assistant professor of general medicine at the University of Michigan Health System, where he is active in patient care and medical education.

Omnigraphics, Inc.

Founded in 1986, Omnigraphics is an independent publisher of respected and authoritative reference books for school, public, and academic libraries. In 1989 they launched the *Health Reference Series* to address a need for comprehensive, up-to-date medical information written for regular people rather than medical professionals. More than 150 volumes later, the critically acclaimed *Health Reference Series*, and related *Teen Health Series*, have become trusted sources for reliable health information. For more information about the company and these series, please visit their website, www.omnigraphics.com.